Vital Statistics for the Public Health Educator

Mark J. Kittleson

Southern Illinois University Press
Carbondale and Edwardsville

Copyright © 1996 by the Board of Trustees,
    Southern Illinois University Press
All rights reserved
Printed in the United States of America

99 98 97 96   4 3 2 1

Library of Congress Cataloging-in-Publication Data

Kittleson, Mark J., date.
    Vital statistics for the public health educator / Mark J. Kittleson.
        p.   cm.
    Includes index.
    1. Medicine—Statistical methods.   2. Public health—Statistical
methods.   3. Statistics, Vital.   I. Title.
    R853.S7K525   1996
    614.4′072—dc20   94-7915
    ISBN 0-8093-1950-0   CIP

The paper used in this publication meets the minimum requirements of American National
Standard for Information Sciences—Permanence of Paper for Printed Library Materials,
ANSI Z39.48-1984. ⊚

To Rachel, for all of her patience,
and to the memory of my father

Contents

Figures

Tables

Acknowledgments

There are many people who should be acknowledged. First, I would like to thank my students who have served as "guinea pigs" in the early drafts of this text. Special thanks to Renee Bleyer and Vera Felts for their comments on these earlier drafts. Second, I would like to thank my colleagues, especially Dale Ritzel, for his support. Third, I would like to thank the people at the Southern Illinois University Press—especially James Simmons and Susan Wilson—for all of their work and support. In addition, special thanks go to Patricia St. John-Doolin for her assistance in the editing of this text. Finally, I would like to thank my family for all of their support.

Vital Statistics for the Public Health Educator

1

An Introduction to Vital Statistics

Welcome to the wonderful world of vital statistics. The ability to interpret and analyze data is of great importance to public health educators located in all types of settings. Unfortunately, public health educators often have had numerous courses in basic and advanced statistics but have received only limited coverage of the practical applications of statistics. Very few public health educators will ever need to do a multivariate analysis, but many will do basic analyses and interpretation of available statistics. Therefore, the purpose of this book is to provide a hands-on approach to the interpretation and reporting of vital statistics.

Definitions

An important part of vital statistics is the understanding of the terminology used. Terms can vary from source to source, and it is very important to know the definition that each source uses. The following are some of the more common terms used in vital statistics:

Demographic data. Characteristics that describe a population make up demographics. By observing such data a public health official can identify certain trends and changes over a period of time. Demographics tend to include not only age and sex but also income, occupation, and utilization of health services (private and public). When coupled with geographical location, these data can be invaluable in planning, assessing, and predicting need. There are numerous sources that can provide demographic data, including both government and nongovernment. A few excellent sources of demographics are the U.S. Census Bureau, marketing reports, and state departments of commerce.

Vital events. Generally speaking, vital events consist of four major activities: births, deaths, marriages, and divorces, all of which are recorded by county and state public health departments. In many states, other events, such as abortions and certain diseases, are also considered "vital" and are likewise recorded.

The U.S. census. As mandated by Congress in 1789, the government canvasses the entire countryside every ten years to ascertain the population of the United States. In spite of several "glitches" during the 1990 event, most experts agree that the census provides the best source of demographic data available to government and public health officials.

The census typically consists of two assessments. The short form is completed by all households and returned to the Census Bureau, while a systematic selection of house-holds determines who completes the long form under the direction of a trained census worker. In the event that the short form is not returned by the requested date, census workers follow up in person. Copies of both the short and long forms can be found in Appendix A.

All data obtained by the census are kept confidential. Yet, when one talks to citizens who do not participate in the census, an underlying theme is a concern for this information being released to unauthorized (or even governmental) officials. In light of the several recent ethical scams involving the government and government officials, one can understand such concern.

The census provides a tremendous amount of information on which government officials can base their allocations of funds and programs. For example, a community's census report of a disproportionately high number of citizens under the age of fifteen might provide the impetus for various government programs to consider funding children's health programs in that community.

Standard Metropolitan Statistical Area (SMSA). Many specific requirements have to be met before an area is classified as a SMSA. One of the major requirements that must be met is that the area must consist of at least fifty thousand residences. In 1980, three hundred and twenty-three such areas were identified. Since then, various political and special interest groups have lobbied to have their region identified as a SMSA. Once identified, the area becomes eligible for certain government programs and more attractive to certain businesses. What appears to have started out as a good idea to assist in planning and identifying metropolitan areas has turned into a political and economic status symbol. As Congress gives more and more exceptions, the concept of a SMSA becomes watered-down.

SMSAs tend to be used by businesses as a key component in their decision whether to build their business at certain locations. Evidentally, such businesses feel that they are at an economic disadvantage to be outside such classifications. In addition, other factors such as certain reimbursements under Medicare/Medicaid tend to be higher in areas designated as SMSAs. Unfortunately, the way that the SMSA system has progressed over the past ten years tends to give the impression that unless an area is designated a SMSA, it is considered to be economically disadvantaged.

In an attempt to offset abuse of the classifications of the SMSA, the government has further broken the SMSA into the Consolidated Metropolitan Statistical Area (CMSA) and the Primary Metropolitan Statistical Area (PMSA). The CMSA is a SMSA that consists of several SMSAs, often cities with millions of residents (Chicago is a good example of a CMSA). The PMSA represent SMSAs where the population is over fifty thousand but typically less than five hundred thousand. Youngstown, Ohio, is an example of a PMSA.

Apgar score. This international code is used to measure the health of an infant. Scores range from zero to ten, with scores lower than eight indicating moderately or severely depressed conditions. Measures occur at one minute and five minutes after birth and identify heart rate, respiratory effort, muscle tone, reflex irritability, and color of skin (e.g., flush, blueness). Although commonly used, the Apgar score is a subjective report, and the final scores depend heavily on the training of the physician in charge.

The Apgar scale was originally developed by a physician, Virginia Apgar, while working as a professor of anesthesiology at New York's Columbia-Presbyterian Medical

Center. The Apgar was developed in the early 1950s, and the name itself coincidentally becomes an acronym for this test: A—stands for appearance (or color); P—pulse; G—grimace or reflex irritability; A—activity or movement; R—respiration.

Live birth. The complete expulsion or extraction of the fetus from its mother constitutes live birth. The fetus must be at least twenty weeks in gestation, and it must show signs of life such as a beating heart, palpitation of the umbilical cord, or definite movement of voluntary muscles.

Premature infant. A premature, or immature, infant is a live-born infant with a birth weight of less than five pounds, eight ounces (2,500 grams), which is sometimes referred to as "low birth weight." Length of gestation is irrelevant in this definition. It is possible for a woman to carry a pregnancy for ten months, and if she delivers a child who weighs less than 2,500 grams, the child would be classified as a premature infant.

Full-term infant. A live-born infant weighing five pounds, eight ounces (2,500 grams), or more, regardless of the length of gestation.

Infant death. Death of a live-born infant occurring within the first year of life.

Neonatal death. Death of a live-born infant occurring within the first twenty-seven days of life. This term can sometimes vary.

Fetal death. Death of a fetus taking place at twenty weeks of gestation or later, and before birth.

Perinatal death. Fetal or neonatal death.

Abortion. Any death of a fetus prior to twenty weeks is considered an abortion. An abortion can be spontaneous, which is a naturally occurring phenomenon, or it can be induced by medical means. These may or may not require reporting to the state for vital records.

Mortality. Death, which is relatively easy to determine. Causes of death are cited in the death certificate.

Morbidity. Illnesses. These data are a little more difficult to gather and in some cases difficult to interpret.

It is very important that the reviewer of vital statistics be aware that definitions may vary; thus, what one state may identify as a neonatal death may be classified as a fetal death in another state. Obviously, such variations need to be kept in mind when interpreting data.

History of Vital Statistics

Vital events are typically births, deaths, marriages, and divorces. State law requires that all vital events be registered, and registration is now quite complete and reliable. Birth certificates serve as proof of citizenship, age, birthplace, and parentage; death certificates are required as burial documents and in the settlement of estates and insurance claims. In the United States, death registration began in Massachusetts in 1857, was extended to ten states, the District of Columbia, and several other cities by 1900, and has been nationwide since 1933. Birth registration began in 1915, encompassing ten states and the District of Columbia. By 1933, all states had been admitted to the nationwide birth and death registration system. A great deal of information is recorded on birth and death certificates. Figures 1.1, 1.2, and 1.3 provide samples of birth and death certificates. Keep in mind though that there are no universal certificates and that each

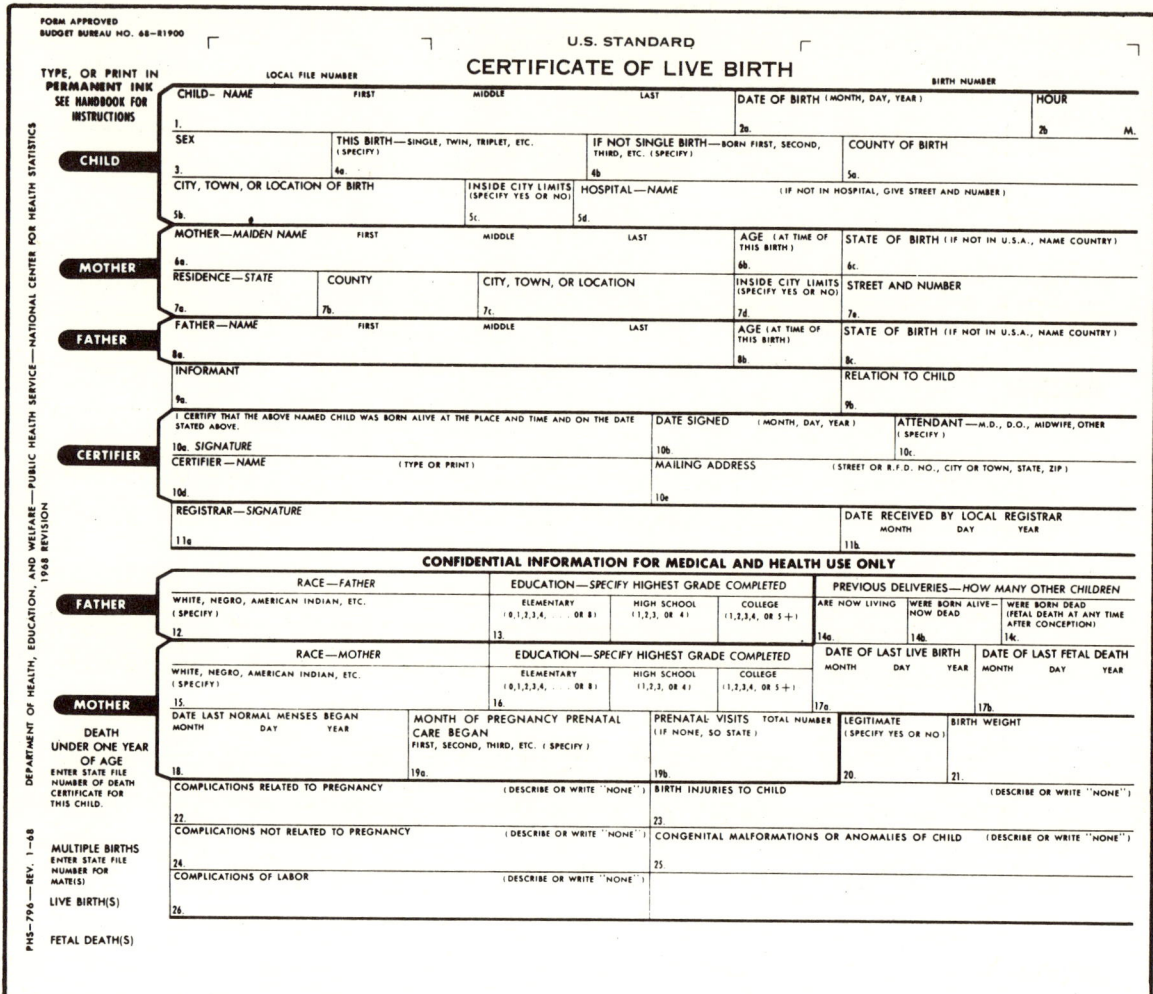

Fig. 1.1. U.S. standard certificate of live birth

state can ask its own particular questions. However, some of the key elements found in a birth certificate include the name; sex; date and time of birth; birth order; weight and length at birth; race of parents; age of parents; place of birth; occupation of father; residence of mother; and physician's (or attendant's) certification. It is also important to keep in mind that there are still many Americans who were born before 1933 who do not have "official" birth certificates.

Besides serving as a source of demographics for vital statisticians, the birth certificate assists the individual in obtaining a social security number and passports, and since the 1986 Immigration Act, serves as proof of citizenship for employment. One can receive a copy of his or her birth certificate by contacting either the state health department or the county health department in the state in which one was born. If it is not

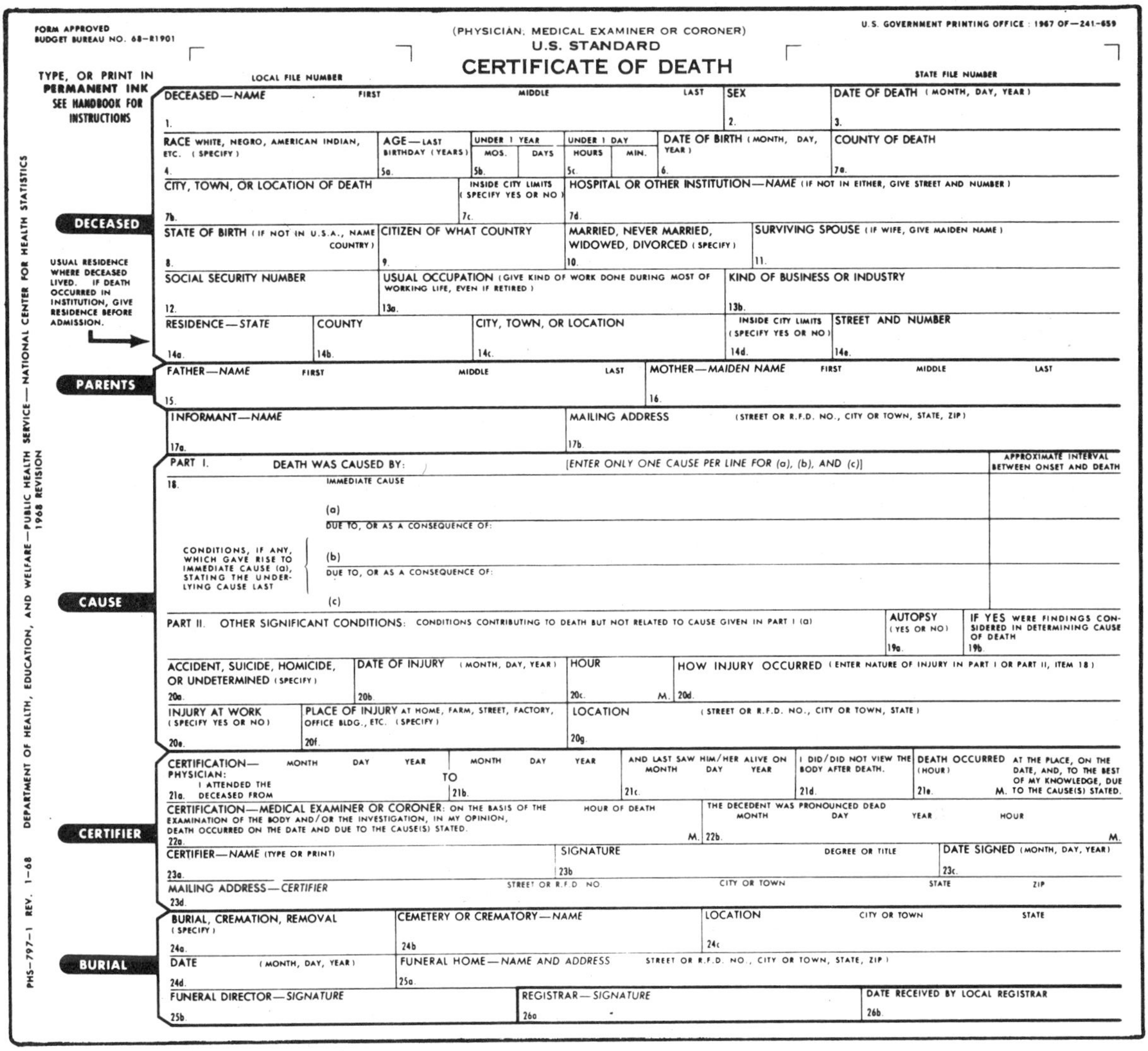

FORM APPROVED
BUDGET BUREAU NO. 68-R1901

(PHYSICIAN, MEDICAL EXAMINER OR CORONER)
U.S. STANDARD
CERTIFICATE OF DEATH

U.S. GOVERNMENT PRINTING OFFICE : 1967 OF—241-659

TYPE, OR PRINT IN PERMANENT INK
SEE HANDBOOK FOR INSTRUCTIONS

LOCAL FILE NUMBER
STATE FILE NUMBER

DECEASED

DECEASED—NAME FIRST MIDDLE LAST 1. | SEX 2. | DATE OF DEATH (MONTH, DAY, YEAR) 3.
RACE WHITE, NEGRO, AMERICAN INDIAN, ETC. (SPECIFY) 4. | AGE—LAST BIRTHDAY (YEARS) 5a. | UNDER 1 YEAR MOS. DAYS 5b. | UNDER 1 DAY HOURS MIN. 5c. | DATE OF BIRTH (MONTH, DAY, YEAR) 6. | COUNTY OF DEATH 7a.
CITY, TOWN, OR LOCATION OF DEATH 7b. | INSIDE CITY LIMITS (SPECIFY YES OR NO) 7c. | HOSPITAL OR OTHER INSTITUTION—NAME (IF NOT IN EITHER, GIVE STREET AND NUMBER) 7d.
STATE OF BIRTH (IF NOT IN U.S.A., NAME COUNTRY) 8. | CITIZEN OF WHAT COUNTRY 9. | MARRIED, NEVER MARRIED, WIDOWED, DIVORCED (SPECIFY) 10. | SURVIVING SPOUSE (IF WIFE, GIVE MAIDEN NAME) 11.
SOCIAL SECURITY NUMBER 12. | USUAL OCCUPATION (GIVE KIND OF WORK DONE DURING MOST OF WORKING LIFE, EVEN IF RETIRED) 13a. | KIND OF BUSINESS OR INDUSTRY 13b.

USUAL RESIDENCE WHERE DECEASED LIVED. IF DEATH OCCURRED IN INSTITUTION, GIVE RESIDENCE BEFORE ADMISSION.

RESIDENCE—STATE 14a. | COUNTY 14b. | CITY, TOWN, OR LOCATION 14c. | INSIDE CITY LIMITS (SPECIFY YES OR NO) 14d. | STREET AND NUMBER 14e.

PARENTS

FATHER—NAME FIRST MIDDLE LAST 15. | MOTHER—MAIDEN NAME FIRST MIDDLE LAST 16.
INFORMANT—NAME 17a. | MAILING ADDRESS (STREET OR R.F.D. NO., CITY OR TOWN, STATE, ZIP) 17b.

CAUSE

PART I. DEATH WAS CAUSED BY: [ENTER ONLY ONE CAUSE PER LINE FOR (a), (b), AND (c)] | APPROXIMATE INTERVAL BETWEEN ONSET AND DEATH
18. IMMEDIATE CAUSE
(a)
DUE TO, OR AS A CONSEQUENCE OF:
CONDITIONS, IF ANY, WHICH GAVE RISE TO IMMEDIATE CAUSE (a), STATING THE UNDERLYING CAUSE LAST
(b)
DUE TO, OR AS A CONSEQUENCE OF:
(c)
PART II. OTHER SIGNIFICANT CONDITIONS: CONDITIONS CONTRIBUTING TO DEATH BUT NOT RELATED TO CAUSE GIVEN IN PART I (a) | AUTOPSY (YES OR NO) 19a. | IF YES WERE FINDINGS CONSIDERED IN DETERMINING CAUSE OF DEATH 19b.
ACCIDENT, SUICIDE, HOMICIDE, OR UNDETERMINED (SPECIFY) 20a. | DATE OF INJURY (MONTH, DAY, YEAR) 20b. | HOUR 20c. M. | HOW INJURY OCCURRED (ENTER NATURE OF INJURY IN PART I OR PART II, ITEM 18) 20d.
INJURY AT WORK (SPECIFY YES OR NO) 20e. | PLACE OF INJURY AT HOME, FARM, STREET, FACTORY, OFFICE BLDG., ETC. (SPECIFY) 20f. | LOCATION (STREET OR R.F.D. NO., CITY OR TOWN, STATE) 20g.

CERTIFIER

CERTIFICATION—PHYSICIAN: I ATTENDED THE DECEASED FROM MONTH DAY YEAR 21a. TO MONTH DAY YEAR 21b. | AND LAST SAW HIM/HER ALIVE ON MONTH DAY YEAR 21c. | I DID/DID NOT VIEW THE BODY AFTER DEATH. 21d. | DEATH OCCURRED (HOUR) 21e. M. AT THE PLACE, ON THE DATE, AND, TO THE BEST OF MY KNOWLEDGE, DUE TO THE CAUSE(S) STATED.
CERTIFICATION—MEDICAL EXAMINER OR CORONER: ON THE BASIS OF THE EXAMINATION OF THE BODY AND/OR THE INVESTIGATION, IN MY OPINION, DEATH OCCURRED ON THE DATE AND DUE TO THE CAUSE(S) STATED. 22a. HOUR OF DEATH M. | THE DECEDENT WAS PRONOUNCED DEAD MONTH DAY YEAR HOUR 22b. M.
CERTIFIER—NAME (TYPE OR PRINT) 23a. | SIGNATURE 23b DEGREE OR TITLE | DATE SIGNED (MONTH, DAY, YEAR) 23c.
MAILING ADDRESS—CERTIFIER 23d. STREET OR R.F.D. NO. CITY OR TOWN STATE ZIP

BURIAL

BURIAL, CREMATION, REMOVAL (SPECIFY) 24a. | CEMETERY OR CREMATORY—NAME 24b | LOCATION CITY OR TOWN STATE 24c
DATE (MONTH, DAY, YEAR) 24d. | FUNERAL HOME—NAME AND ADDRESS STREET OR R.F.D. NO., CITY OR TOWN, STATE, ZIP 25a.
FUNERAL DIRECTOR—SIGNATURE 25b. | REGISTRAR—SIGNATURE 26a | DATE RECEIVED BY LOCAL REGISTRAR 26b.

DEPARTMENT OF HEALTH, EDUCATION, AND WELFARE—PUBLIC HEALTH SERVICE—NATIONAL CENTER FOR HEALTH STATISTICS
1968 REVISION
PHS-797-1 REV. 1-68

Fig. 1.2. U.S. standard certificate of death

possible to obtain the birth certificate from either of these places, they should be able to provide information on who to contact.

Death certificates typically include the name; date and time of death; race; age; place of birth; names of decedent's parents; name and address of survivor (or informant); marital status; occupation; place of residence; cause(s) of death; place of death; burial data; death due to injury: accident, suicide, or homicide; physician's (or coroner's) certificate.

It should be pointed out that public health officials depend greatly on the efforts of many people to maintain vital records. Physicians, hospital personnel, funeral directors,

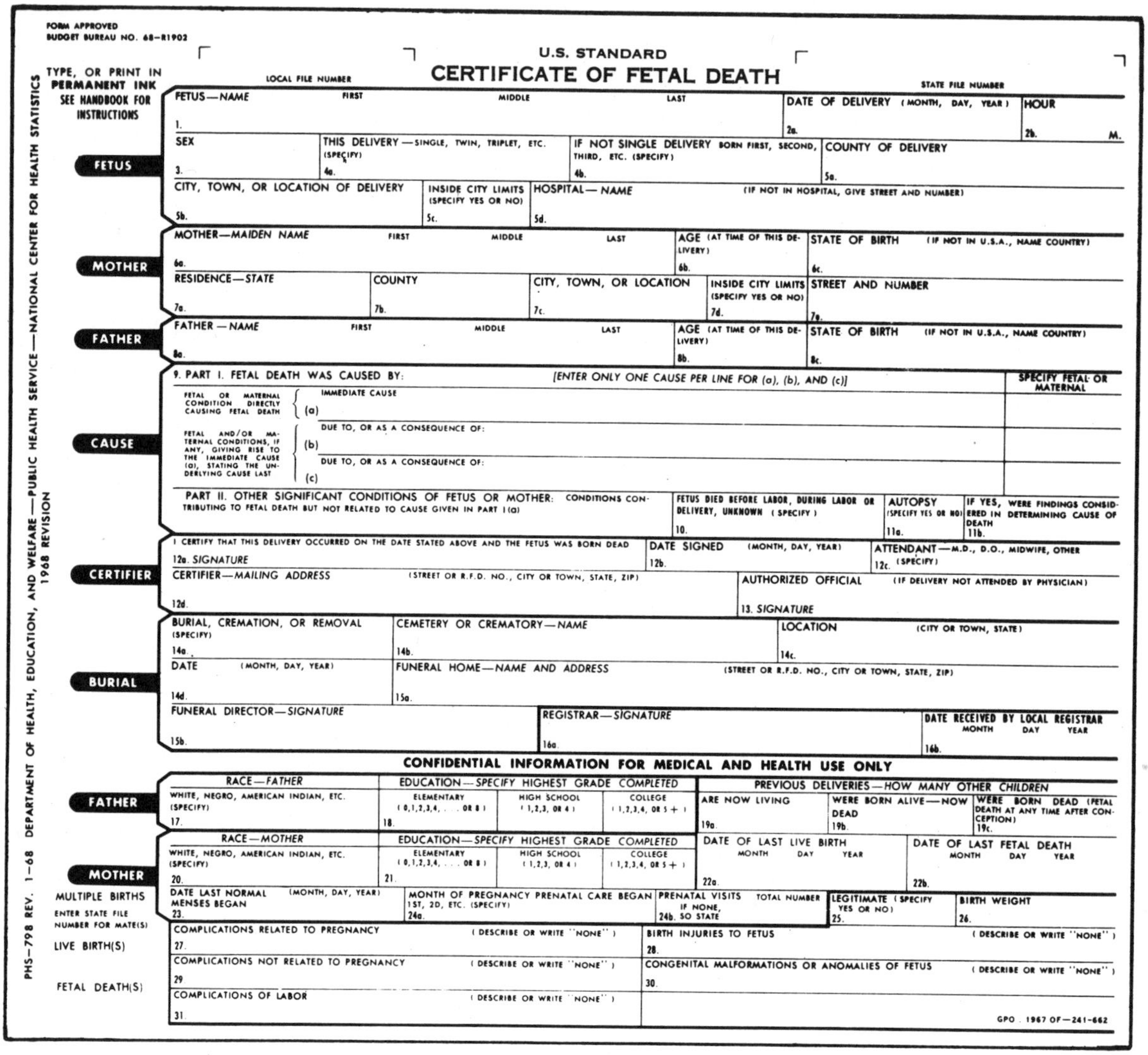

FORM APPROVED
BUDGET BUREAU NO. 68–R1902

PHS–798 REV. 1–68 DEPARTMENT OF HEALTH, EDUCATION, AND WELFARE—PUBLIC HEALTH SERVICE—NATIONAL CENTER FOR HEALTH STATISTICS
1968 REVISION

TYPE, OR PRINT IN PERMANENT INK
SEE HANDBOOK FOR INSTRUCTIONS

LOCAL FILE NUMBER — U.S. STANDARD CERTIFICATE OF FETAL DEATH — STATE FILE NUMBER

FETUS
1. FETUS—NAME FIRST MIDDLE LAST
2a. DATE OF DELIVERY (MONTH, DAY, YEAR)
2b. HOUR M.
3. SEX
4a. THIS DELIVERY—SINGLE, TWIN, TRIPLET, ETC. (SPECIFY)
4b. IF NOT SINGLE DELIVERY BORN FIRST, SECOND, THIRD, ETC. (SPECIFY)
5a. COUNTY OF DELIVERY
5b. CITY, TOWN, OR LOCATION OF DELIVERY
5c. INSIDE CITY LIMITS (SPECIFY YES OR NO)
5d. HOSPITAL—NAME (IF NOT IN HOSPITAL, GIVE STREET AND NUMBER)

MOTHER
6a. MOTHER—MAIDEN NAME FIRST MIDDLE LAST
6b. AGE (AT TIME OF THIS DELIVERY)
6c. STATE OF BIRTH (IF NOT IN U.S.A., NAME COUNTRY)
7a. RESIDENCE—STATE
7b. COUNTY
7c. CITY, TOWN, OR LOCATION
7d. INSIDE CITY LIMITS (SPECIFY YES OR NO)
7e. STREET AND NUMBER

FATHER
8a. FATHER—NAME FIRST MIDDLE LAST
8b. AGE (AT TIME OF THIS DELIVERY)
8c. STATE OF BIRTH (IF NOT IN U.S.A., NAME COUNTRY)

CAUSE
9. PART I. FETAL DEATH WAS CAUSED BY: [ENTER ONLY ONE CAUSE PER LINE FOR (a), (b), AND (c)] — SPECIFY FETAL OR MATERNAL
FETAL OR MATERNAL CONDITION DIRECTLY CAUSING FETAL DEATH (a) IMMEDIATE CAUSE
FETAL AND/OR MATERNAL CONDITIONS, IF ANY, GIVING RISE TO THE IMMEDIATE CAUSE (a), STATING THE UNDERLYING CAUSE LAST (b) DUE TO, OR AS A CONSEQUENCE OF: (c) DUE TO, OR AS A CONSEQUENCE OF:
PART II. OTHER SIGNIFICANT CONDITIONS OF FETUS OR MOTHER: CONDITIONS CONTRIBUTING TO FETAL DEATH BUT NOT RELATED TO CAUSE GIVEN IN PART I (a)
10. FETUS DIED BEFORE LABOR, DURING LABOR OR DELIVERY, UNKNOWN (SPECIFY)
11a. AUTOPSY (SPECIFY YES OR NO)
11b. IF YES, WERE FINDINGS CONSIDERED IN DETERMINING CAUSE OF DEATH

CERTIFIER
I CERTIFY THAT THIS DELIVERY OCCURRED ON THE DATE STATED ABOVE AND THE FETUS WAS BORN DEAD
12a. SIGNATURE
12b. DATE SIGNED (MONTH, DAY, YEAR)
12c. ATTENDANT—M.D., D.O., MIDWIFE, OTHER (SPECIFY)
12d. CERTIFIER—MAILING ADDRESS (STREET OR R.F.D. NO., CITY OR TOWN, STATE, ZIP)
13. AUTHORIZED OFFICIAL (IF DELIVERY NOT ATTENDED BY PHYSICIAN) SIGNATURE

BURIAL
14a. BURIAL, CREMATION, OR REMOVAL (SPECIFY)
14b. CEMETERY OR CREMATORY—NAME
14c. LOCATION (CITY OR TOWN, STATE)
14d. DATE (MONTH, DAY, YEAR)
15a. FUNERAL HOME—NAME AND ADDRESS (STREET OR R.F.D. NO., CITY OR TOWN, STATE, ZIP)
15b. FUNERAL DIRECTOR—SIGNATURE
16a. REGISTRAR—SIGNATURE
16b. DATE RECEIVED BY LOCAL REGISTRAR MONTH DAY YEAR

CONFIDENTIAL INFORMATION FOR MEDICAL AND HEALTH USE ONLY

FATHER
17. RACE—FATHER WHITE, NEGRO, AMERICAN INDIAN, ETC. (SPECIFY)
18. EDUCATION—SPECIFY HIGHEST GRADE COMPLETED ELEMENTARY (0,1,2,3,4, . . . OR 8) HIGH SCHOOL (1,2,3, OR 4) COLLEGE (1,2,3,4, OR 5 +)
PREVIOUS DELIVERIES—HOW MANY OTHER CHILDREN
19a. ARE NOW LIVING
19b. WERE BORN ALIVE—NOW DEAD
19c. WERE BORN DEAD (FETAL DEATH AT ANY TIME AFTER CONCEPTION)

MOTHER
20. RACE—MOTHER WHITE, NEGRO, AMERICAN INDIAN, ETC. (SPECIFY)
21. EDUCATION—SPECIFY HIGHEST GRADE COMPLETED ELEMENTARY (0,1,2,3,4, . . . OR 8) HIGH SCHOOL (1,2,3, OR 4) COLLEGE (1,2,3,4, OR 5 +)
22a. DATE OF LAST LIVE BIRTH MONTH DAY YEAR
22b. DATE OF LAST FETAL DEATH MONTH DAY YEAR

MULTIPLE BIRTHS ENTER STATE FILE NUMBER FOR MATE(S)
LIVE BIRTH(S)
FETAL DEATH(S)

23. DATE LAST NORMAL MENSES BEGAN (MONTH, DAY, YEAR)
24a. MONTH OF PREGNANCY PRENATAL CARE BEGAN 1ST, 2D, ETC. (SPECIFY)
24b. PRENATAL VISITS TOTAL NUMBER IF NONE, SO STATE
25. LEGITIMATE (SPECIFY YES OR NO)
26. BIRTH WEIGHT
27. COMPLICATIONS RELATED TO PREGNANCY (DESCRIBE OR WRITE "NONE")
28. BIRTH INJURIES TO FETUS (DESCRIBE OR WRITE "NONE")
29. COMPLICATIONS NOT RELATED TO PREGNANCY (DESCRIBE OR WRITE "NONE")
30. CONGENITAL MALFORMATIONS OR ANOMALIES OF FETUS (DESCRIBE OR WRITE "NONE")
31. COMPLICATIONS OF LABOR (DESCRIBE OR WRITE "NONE")

GPO . 1967 OF—241-662

Fig. 1.3. U.S. standard certificate of fetal death

coroners, and medical examiners finalize data that are sent to various local and state public health departments.

The National Center for Health Statistics collects a systematic sampling of 10 percent of the births and deaths in each state. From this, it publishes the monthly *Vital Statistics Report*. Annually, it issues the four-volume *Vital Statistics of the United States*, which includes many detailed tables on vital events for all sorts of demographic characteristics and for major geographical subdivisions. Data on marriages and divorces are similarly collected and published in a separate volume of *Vital Statistics of the United States*. All such information is found in any government depository library.

All states are now compiling computerized death certificate data, or "death tapes," which are computer-readable extracts of the most important data appearing on death certificates. Since 1979, the National Center for Health Statistics has prepared the *National Death Index*, a nationwide, computerized index of death records compiled from tapes submitted by the vital statistics offices of each state. These tapes contain a standard set of identifying data for each decedent. The *Index* permits researchers to determine if persons in their studies have died. For each such case, the death certificate is available, along with the identity of the state where the death occurred and the date of death. Given these mortality data, the researcher can order a copy of the death certificate from the state's vital statistics office. Confidentiality of data is guaranteed by law.

This collection of vital statistics is incredibly important in aiding public health efforts to plan programs. As personal computers become increasingly cheaper and more popular to use, a whole new public health effort can soon be underway. In Illinois, my colleagues here at Southern Illinois University along with the Illinois Department of Public Health have developed the Illinois Project for Local Assessment of Needs (IPLAN), which combines vital statistics from all counties and communities in the state and which can easily be loaded onto a personal computer. It takes approximately ten megabytes of hard-disk space to hold the data for just 1990, and plans are in the works to add data for each subsequent year. To operate most efficiently, a 386-model computer (preferably a 486) is needed. The menu-driven IPLAN data system contains both county and community data and has the capability to group counties or communities, provide classifications by race, ethnicity, gender, and age, calculate data into rates, provide United States and Year 2000 Objectives, and be outputed onto a printout.

Computer "bulletin boards" are also increasing throughout the United States. A modem is necessary to join the network as well as the payment of a monthly service fee and on-line charge. CompuServe is one of the most popular systems and is available in many sites throughout the country. CompuServe can provide demographics to the vital statistician, often with specific county information.

Besides the information from the census or from vital statistics, additional major data systems are available for public health educators from the National Center for Health Statistics. The following major data systems are listed in Sandra Surber-Smith's 1981 article "Major Data Systems of the National Center for Health Statistics" in *Public Health Reports* (vol. 96 [3]: 200–201).

- The National Natality Survey compiles data on socioeconomic and demographic characteristics of mothers, prenatal care, pregnancy history, occupational background, and the health status of mothers and infants. The data are collected from periodic surveys mailed to new mothers.
- The National Health Interview Survey focuses primarily on health conditions and factors about American's health, asking questions regarding the incidence of illnesses and injuries, prevalence of chronic diseases, and other health-related topics, such as physician, dentist, and hospital visits.
- The National Health and Nutrition Examination Survey began in 1959 and has continued to take place every two to four years. It assesses clinical data such as blood pressure, serum cholesterol, visual acuity, and nutritional status and deficiencies.
- The National Ambulatory Medical Care Survey is analogous to the National Health and Nutrition Examination Survey. This survey reviews the records of approximately fifty thousand visits to physicians' offices and requests information on diagnoses and symptoms identified in such visits.

- The National Hospital Discharge Survey, begun in 1965, samples approximately two hundred thousand hospital records, reviewing diagnoses, surgeries, and various characteristics of patients and correlating these factors to the size and location of the various hospitals.
- The National Mortality Survey reviews data on various socioeconomic characteristics, facilities used, costs incurred, and related health factors occurring during a patient's last year of life.
- The National Nursing Home Survey, begun in 1963, compiles data on nursing homes, their services, and the characteristics of the residents.
- The National Medical Care Utilization and Expenditures Survey reviews the use of and expenditures for health services during the previous year, collecting the data from household interviews.
- The National Inventory of Family Planning Service Sites lists all clinics that provide family planning services. The information is based on data collected in questionnaires sent to such facilities.
- The National Master Facility Inventory lists inpatient health facilities in the United States. It also identifies services, location, and staff in each of these facilities.
- The Health Professions Survey identifies information on the number, location, training, and specialization of primary and allied health professionals.
- The National Reporting System for Family Planning Services collects data on persons receiving medical family planning services. Data are collected from clinic records for patients at federally supported family planning programs, as well as other public and private organizations.

Besides the federal government, there are other sources that the public health educator may want to review when looking at planning programs. Vital statistics are important, but they do not always explain why events occur. Other information such as housing, incomes, occupations, cost of living, and educational levels may assist in identifying and/or explaining reasons for certain trends measured by the vital statistics.

Marketing research can also be an important source of demographics. Major corporations spend millions of dollars trying to get people to buy their products. Before they invest their money, they must develop a marketing strategy that will give them the biggest "bang" for their dollar. Thus, it is important for such corporations to understand the people they are trying to target for their products.

Reference books that may contain useful information for your state are John Clements's books. Clements has written books on several states and includes a county by county assessment of information that can be of relevance to the public health educator. For example, this book will include death rates of various age groups, birthrates among various race and/or ethnic groups, or types of illnesses the county is experiencing. Your local library may carry these books. The book on Illinois is entitled *A Comprehensive Look at Illinois Today County by County. Flying the Colors: Illinois Facts* (Dallas, TX: Clements Research II).

Finally, there are numerous software programs that can be of assistance. PCUSA and US Atlas are available commercially and can provide information at national, state, and local levels. US Atlas contains county, state, and national information that might be relevant to the public health educator. Such information includes birthrates and death rates. In addition to these commercially available sources, many libraries are now carrying the entire census on CD-ROM, which is available for a nominal fee.

2

Understanding Basic Statistics

Fortunately with the use of computers and calculators one can forego the basics of many statistical analyses. With that pressure off, it's important for the vital statistician or public health educator to become familiar with the types of data that they will be using. As I mentioned before, there will be very few times in your life that you will be running a multiple linear regression for your worksite. Yet many of you will be looking at basic correlations, comparisons between groups, or other relatively simple processes. This chapter is an introduction to some very basic terms and applications of statistics. As both a practitioner and a consumer, you need to be able to identify inappropriate usages of statistics. If you are feeling hesitant about your basic math skills, this might be a good time for you to review the basic math skills presented in Appendix D.

Data

Data, or representative numbers can be classified into one of four types (by the way, the word *data* is plural and should be reflected as such in your writing. If you have trouble with this, do as I do: every time I see the word *data*, I think of the word *cows*; it makes it easier to use the proper grammatical forms).

Nominal data. Nominal data, the simplest type, are used for description and identification purposes only. Nominal data do not reflect good or bad, better or worse, or wrong or right.

An example of nominal data is the use of numbers on professional ball players. In football, numbers on the players may represent a certain position that is played (e.g., the numbers 1 to 19 are typically reserved for quarterbacks). The numbering of football player X as number 89 and football player Y as number 22 doesn't mean that player X is better than player Y.

Nominal data are used extensively in vital statistics. For example, the classification of an individual as male or female is an example of nominal data. The race of the individual is another example. Neither indicate right or wrong, better or worse, or good or bad. This type of data should be considered very important and useful.

Ordinal data. Ordinal data, besides serving as description, can also serve as a ranking mechanism. Ranking your top ten teachers is an example of the use of ordinal data. Another example that's relevant to vital statistics is the classification of a person's income into a series of categories such as high, medium, or low. Obviously, those in the high category make more money than the other two, but you do not know how much more. That is one of the limitations of ordinal data—all it can do is rank (and classify).

Going back to ranking your top ten teachers, with ordinal data all you have is that top ten list—you do not have the degree of comparison between the first person and the tenth person. Perhaps your first choice is far superior to the other nine; maybe the second through tenth choices were just a toss-up. Such information is not reflected in ordinal data. This does not make it poor data, but it is restricted.

Interval data and ratio data. Interval data and ratio data can not only serve as classification (like nominal data) and ranking data (like ordinal data) but can also provide some sense of distance between each bit of data. Interval data are singular in that a true zero does not exist in these data. For example, a thermometer reading is an example of interval data. When it's zero out, it doesn't mean we have no temperature, it means it's cold outside. Also, when the temperature drops from eighty degrees to seventy degrees or from twenty degrees to ten degrees, both have a drop of ten degrees.

On the other hand, ratio data do exhibit a true zero, so ratio data encompass all of the types of data described here. For the sake of argument and ease of understanding, this text will use interval and ratio data interchangeably (which should make some true statisticians gag). Really, though, there is little difference between interval data and ratio data for the vital statistician/public health educator.

Another example of interval/ratio data can be shown in comparison of ages. A person who is seventy is twice as old as someone who is thirty-five. And some people would question whether a person ever has no age (a true zero). White blood cell counts is another example of the use of interval/ratio data and the confusion that sometimes occurs between the two (and why I just combine the two together). Is it possible to have zero white blood cells, or are you dead at that time? Nonetheless, the increase from ten thousand to fifteen thousand white blood cells is an understandable and measurable term.

Any interval/ratio data can be converted to ordinal data. The measure of income is interval/ratio data. Yet, if you were to dichotomize the data into high, medium, and low categories, that data would be considered ordinal. If you have ever taken a survey where you were asked to state your age, you have given the researcher datum that is considered to be interval/ratio. However, if you responded to a question about age by checking a box similar to this example, the datum you gave would be considered ordinal.

Age:
_____ 18–22
_____ 23–27
_____ 28–35
_____ 36–49
_____ 50 and above

Certainly, anyone checking the 50 and above category is older than the rest, but the researcher cannot tell how much older the person is than someone in the 36–49 category. Perhaps this person just turned fifty two days ago, and this person's spouse is still forty-nine but turns fifty tomorrow. Technically they are in separate categories, when in reality they are only three days apart in age. That's one of the drawbacks of using ordinal data.

A few examples of some types of sources of data follow. Take a few minutes and indicate which of these would produce nominal, ordinal, or interval/ratio data.

age
income
sex
race
marital status
blood glucose levels
number of children
birth order of children
socioeconomic status

Of the examples above, the sources that would supply only nominal data are marital status, sex, and race. Those items that exhibit ordinal data are birth order of children and socioeconomic status, and those that are considered interval/ratio data sources would include age, income, blood glucose levels, and number of children.

Data Analysis

Pity the poor vital statisticians who had to compute the data by hand. Fortunately, because of the advent of computers and calculators, we don't have to suffer that fate. Yet it is important to understand the concepts behind these data analyses. You'll never have to do it by hand (unless you have a lot of extra time), but you will probably run analyses at certain times throughout your professional life.

Depending on the type of data you have, you will be limited as to the type of analysis you use. Three of the most basic analyses are the mean, median, and mode. Let's talk about the mode first.

The *mode* is the most commonly cited variable. For example, if you were to ask how much money the students in your class had in their pocket at the present time, you'd find a wide range of amounts. The mode is the most often cited figure. For the sake of argument, let's say that there are nine students in your class, plus your professor, and the range of money is as follows:

Student A $20
Student B $10
Student C $30
Student D $10
Student E $10
Student F $90
Student G $10
Student H $20
Student I $20
Professor $ 1

Of these figures, which is the mode? The most often cited figure is $10, so the mode is 10.

$$
\begin{array}{|c|}
\hline
5 \\
4 \\
4 \\
3 \\
2 \\
2 \\
2 \\
\hline
\end{array}
$$

Fig. 2.1. Median of odd numbers

The *mean* is the arithmetic average of the total. To get this figure, you add the entire column and divide by the number of entrants. If you were to total the above column, it would come to 221. Since you have 10 people, you divide 221 by 10, and your mean is $22.10. Thus, the average amount of money that the fellow residents in your class have in their pockets at the time of this survey is $22.10.

Finally, the *median* is another way to help describe the monetary factors of this group. The median is the halfway point, where 50% of the numbers are above and 50% are below. This is a little more difficult to ascertain. It is easier if you have an odd number of entrants, because you can just pick the middle number.

Of the numbers in figure 2.1, which one lies where half of the scores are above and half are below? Since there are seven numbers, all you need to do is to count up four or down four. The resulting median number is 3.

What is the median of the four scores in figure 2.2? If you go up two (half of the total of four) and if you go down two you come to a dead end. When you need to find the median of an even number of groups, you need to average out the two closest middle figures. In this case, 3 + 2 ÷ 2 = 2.5. So the median of 4, 3, 2, and 1 is 2.5. That is the median number in which 50% of the numbers are above and 50% of the numbers are below.

Now let's go back to our earlier study of the money in your classroom. The first thing you need to do to find the median amount is to list the money in declining order:

Student F	$90
Student C	$30
Student A	$20
Student H	$20
Student I	$20
Student B	$10
Student D	$10
Student E	$10
Student G	$10
Professor	$ 1

Since there are ten subjects, you can figure out that 5 is somewhere near the median. So count up and down five, and you will be between student I and student B. Since you have an even number, you need to add the amounts of students I and B and divide by 2.

```
4
3
2
1
```

Fig. 2.2. Median of even numbers

Thus, the median of this group is 15—this is where 50% of the group is above and 50% of the group is below. So the three key statistics for this study are mode—$10; mean—$22.10; and median—$15. Note that although all three are different they can each help describe the population under study.

When you look at these numbers, it appears that there are great discrepancies between the three, but they are expressing totally different ideas. For example, the mean attempts to balance things out. If that one student hadn't had $90, the mean would have dropped dramatically. Try figuring out the mean without student F. The total is 131 ÷ 9, which equals $14.56.

Every so often we hear the government report on the "average" income for the United States. They use the three figures computed by mode, mean, and median analyses, but many officials "abuse" these terms terribly. For example, they report that the mean salary is $30,000. Keep in mind that they are adding together the entire population's salary and dividing by the number of the population. So your salary is being added in along with H. Ross Perot's. The same government report will indicate that the mode (most frequently reported salary) is $18,000 and that the median (where half of all salaries are above and half are below) is $23,000.

Mode, Median, Mean, and Data Classification

The type of data (i.e., nominal, ordinal, interval/ratio) limits the vital statistician in the analysis of the data. For example, let's imagine you have nominal (classification) data. You have a football team with each player having a separate number. Now, would it make sense to add all of the numbers and divide by the number of players to get a mean number? This, as you may recall, is the arithematic mean analysis. Let's say that this arithematic mean is 38.6. What would 38.6 mean? It doesn't mean a thing. Thus, it is not a good idea to do a mean on nominal data. So what analysis would be appropriate for nominal data? Before we answer that, let's think of a typical nominal datum that might occur in the public health field.

A common classification is based on a person's sex. People are either males or females. There is no one sex that is better or worse; one is just classified as either male or female. Oftentimes, vital statisticians will identify males as 1 and females as 2 (or vice versa). Let's imagine that you have 15 males and 25 females. It wouldn't make sense to add up all of those 1s and 2s and divide by 40 (the total number of people). You'd get some number like 1.75. What would that mean? Nothing. The statistics methods that you would probably employ would be frequencies and percentages.

When you have ordinal data, you can use frequencies and percentages, but you also can use median analysis. For example, let's say that you have a question on a survey that requests the following information:

I think this book is great.
a. strongly agree
b. agree
c. don't know
d. disagree
e. strongly disagree

We've all answered questions like this. What type of data is this? In spite of the fact that researchers have arbitrarily assigned numbers to it (i.e., a = 5, b = 4, c = 3, d = 2, e = 1), it is actually only ordinal data. So because it is ordinal data, you are limited in the type of statistical analysis that you can run. You can do frequencies and percentages and a test for the mode (the most frequently reported answer). You could also do a median (which answers had 50% of the respondents above and which had 50% below). If you wanted to determine if there was any significance you could run a chi-square, which I discuss later in this chapter.

When you have interval/ratio data, you can use the mode, median, and arithmetic mean analyses. For example, suppose you have income as a variable and it is reported in dollars. Of your sample (let's say you have the incomes of 10,000 people), you could figure the most commonly reported income (mode); you could see what income had 50% above and 50% below (median); or you could add all of the incomes together and divide by 10,000 to get the arithematic mean. If you wanted to see if there was a difference between two groups (e.g., males and females), you could run a test of means (explained later in this chapter), because this data is considered interval/ratio.

Range and Standard Deviation

To further describe the population in your study, you may want to include the *range* of moneys. Subtract the lowest amount of money, $1 (this, as you may not know, is typical of most professors), from the highest amount, $90, to find the money range, which is $89. Range calculation works for small amounts or for a limited number of subjects, but it is a little impractical for anything of any large scale. For example, what is the range of salary in the United States? H. Ross Perot's $2.5 billion salary minus the lowest income in the country, say a professor's at $12, gives us a range of $2,499,999,988.

To aid us in calculating ranges of larger figures or groups, we can use another analyzing device called the *standard deviation*. The standard deviation (SD) is used to give an *average* variable range of a group of data. In order to understand this, we have to talk theory.

Theoretically speaking, in a "normal" population we would have some poor people, some rich people, and a large group of people in the middle. This concept would form a curve such as the one in figure 2.3.

To help us in analyzing this data, statisticians grid the curve into standard deviations. Typically, there are three standard deviations above the mean (the middle, or the peak, of the curve) and three standard deviations below the mean. In a perfect curve, if you go one standard deviation above and one standard deviation below the mean, you'll encompass about 67% of the total group. If you go two standard deviations above and

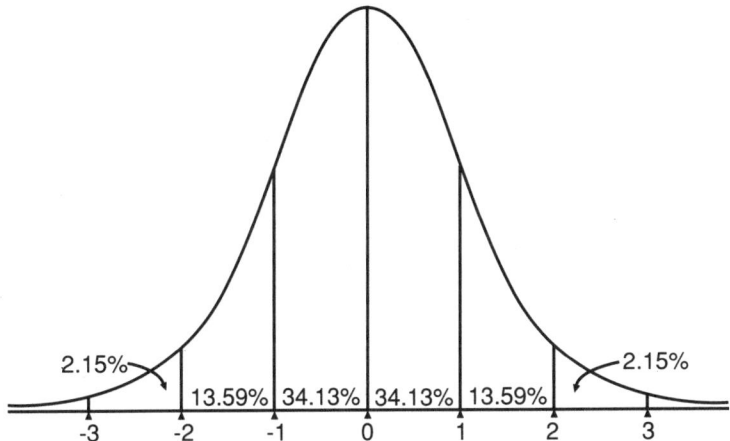

Fig. 2.3. Standard normal curve of a population

below the mean, you'll include about 95%. If you go three standard deviations above and below the mean, you'll encompass about 99% of the group. Thus, an important formula to remember is:

$$\text{Mean} \pm 1 \text{ SD} = 68.26\%$$
$$\text{Mean} \pm 2 \text{ SD} = 95.45\%$$
$$\text{Mean} \pm 3 \text{ SD} = 99.74\%$$

Now, let's imagine that you surveyed a group of individuals to find their annual incomes and you then divided them into females and males. Your survey leads to the following two curves shown in figures 2.4 and 2.5.

As you can see, the curve of the males is a little flatter than the curve of the females. Does this mean anything? Yes, it means quite a bit. Let's take this a few steps further.

The males' mean income is $20,000, whereas the females' mean income is also $20,000. Based on that statistic it appears that both groups are very similar. They both average $20,000 income. Well, remember earlier when we talked about how the mean, mode, and median can all be different? Look at the curves. You can see that the male curve is flatter. The "distribution" of the males' incomes appears to be different than that of the females'.

Let's say that the standard deviation of income on this curve for males is $5,000. So, according to the calculations, approximately 68% of the males' annual incomes fall between $15,000 and $25,000 (remember: mean ± 1 SD = 68.26%). Approximately 95.5% of all males had annual incomes between $10,000 and $30,000, and nearly 99.7% had annual incomes between $5,000 and $35,000. Less than 1% of the males had incomes less than $5,000 and more than $35,000.

Now, for the females, let's say that the standard deviation is $2,500. Once again, you can see that approximately 68% of the females had annual incomes between $17,500 and $22,500 (mean ± 1 SD = 68.26%); 95.5% of the females had an income between $15,000 and $25,000, and 99.7% of the females had incomes between $12,500

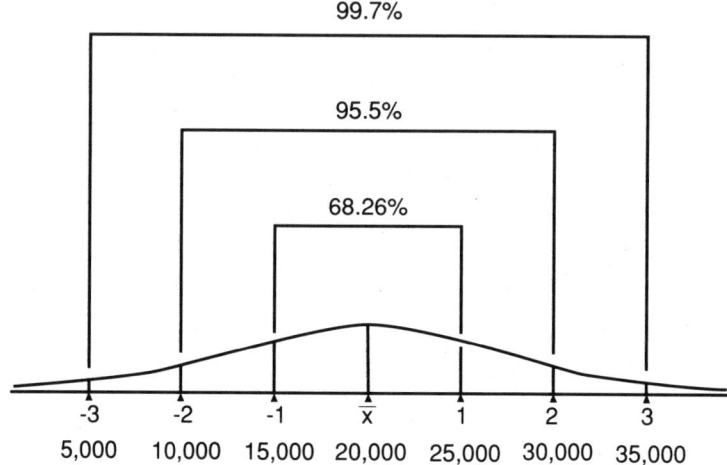

Fig. 2.4. Curve showing standard deviation of males' annual income

and $27,500. Less than 1% of the females had incomes either below $12,500 or above $27,500.

Now, look at these two curves and the numbers. First, let's see what these numbers mean. What can you tell me about the range and variability of the incomes of males and females? Well, I hope you will note that there appears to be a wider range of incomes among males than among females. Females' incomes tend to cluster more around the middle of the curve. This is a very important concept. The standard deviation can help you tell a lot about the variability of the group you are reviewing. Now, look again at the two figures. Remember, the males' curve is flatter, indicating that there is a wider variability between members of the group. The smaller the standard deviation, the more *similar* or *homogenous* the group and the bigger the bulge in the curve. The larger the standard deviation, the more *different* the group and the flatter the curve.

These very simple approaches to describing a population can be called *descriptive statistics*. They may seem simple, but they are nonetheless very important. Oftentimes people sneer at descriptive statistics (typically those individuals who eat, sleep, and drink statistics), but they serve a very important function. In many instances, the vital statistician will need to use descriptive statistics for their reports.

Besides being able to perform such analyses, you need to be able to understand the general concepts and terms of analyses. Since you are not only a practitioner but also a consumer of research and vital statistics, you need to know some other basic techniques. It is important that you understand correlations, significance, chi-square and test of means analyses, and analysis of variance.

Correlation

Correlations look at relationships between events, groups, or other data. A relationship often makes people think that one event causes the other to occur. That isn't necessarily the case. For example, a fellow colleague of mine indicated that whenever he had to pay his six-month premium for auto insurance, he noticed a higher incidence

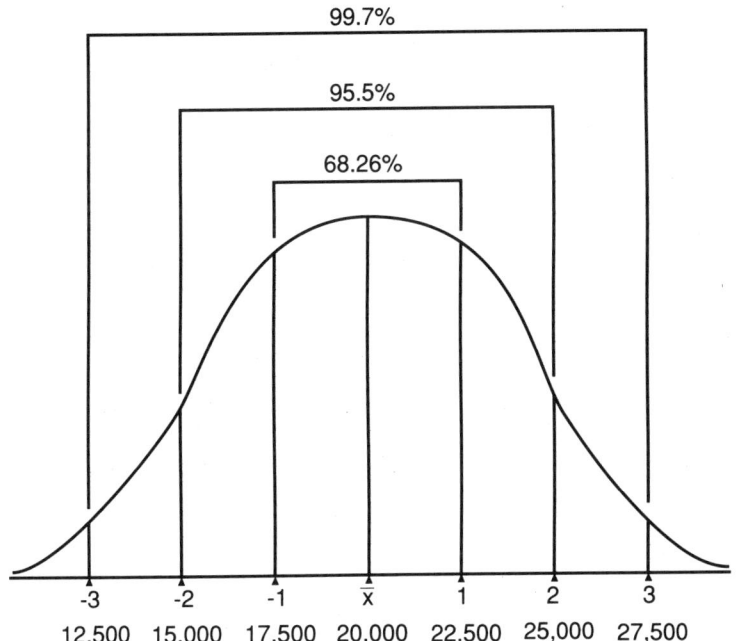

Fig. 2.5. Curve showing standard deviation of females' annual income

of suicide among students at our university. He happens to pay his premiums in November and May. Now does the payment of his automobile insurance cause this increase in suicides? No, but there *appears* to be a correlation. A correlational study merely determines whether there is a relationship between two items. It is up to the researchers to ascertain whether it is a causal relationship. This premise is very important to remember—a correlation merely measures a relationship; it does not determine cause and effect. The pickle eating article in figure 2.6 illustrates how relationships can be taken to extremes.

So if your purpose is to measure a relationship, what should you know about it? Well, first of all you can either have a perfect positive correlation or a perfect negative correlation. Perfect correlations are 1.00 and −1.00 respectively. We don't have too many perfect correlations anywhere. A *positive correlation* occurs when both components of a relationship move in the same direction. For example, a well-known positive correlation exists between education and income. It's true that one can make a lot of money without going to school, but overall it appears that the more education one receives, the more money one will make (with the possible exception of university faculty). But one does not necessarily cause the other to increase.

A *negative correlation* is evident when the components move in opposite directions. For example, when one's income increases, the less taxes one pays (no, I'm just kidding on this one, I think). A negative correlation might be exhibited when inflation in the United States goes up and the president's approval rating goes down.

The closer one gets to either a +1.00 or a −1.00, the stronger the relationship. It is useful to identify such relationships because they can lead to a series of questions for researchers to help them predict or investigate such instances.

Evils of Pickle Eating
Everett D. Edington

Pickles are associated with all the major diseases of the body. Eating them breeds war and Communism. They can be related to most airline tragedies. Auto accidents are caused by pickles. There exists a positive relationship between crime waves and consumption of this fruit of the cucurbit family. For example . . .

Nearly all sick people have eaten pickles. The effects are obviously cumulative:

- 99.9% of all people who die from cancer have eaten pickles.
- 100% of all soldiers have eaten pickles.
- 96.8% of all Communist sympathizers have eaten pickles.
- 99.7% of the people involved in air and auto accidents ate pickles within 14 days preceding the accident.
- 93.1% of juvenile delinquents come from homes where pickles are served frequently. Evidence points to the long-term effects of pickle eating.
- Of the people born in 1839 who later dined on pickles, there has been a 100% mortality.

All pickle eaters born between 1849 and 1859 have wrinkled skin, have lost most of their teeth, have brittle bones and failing eyesight—if the ills of pickle eating have not already caused their death.

Even more convincing is the report of a noted team of medical specialists: rats force-fed with 20 pounds of pickles per day for 30 days developed bulging abdomens. Their appetites for Wholesome food were destroyed.

In spite of all the evidence, pickle growers and packers continue to spread their evil. More than 120,000 acres of fertile U.S. soil are devoted to growing pickles. Our per capital consumption is nearly four pounds.

Eat orchid petal soup. Practically no one has as many problems from eating orchid petal soup as they do with eating pickles.

Fig. 2.6. Example of spurious association (from "Evils of Pickle Eating," by Everett D. Edington, originally printed in *Cyanograms*)

One of the most common measurements of correlations is the Pearson Product Coefficiency Correlation. The Pearson Product uses the letter r to identify it's relationship. Below is the formula, but quite frankly, if you ever decide to figure a correlation by hand, you should probably talk to your physician and get a referral for a good psychiatrist.

Formula for computing Pearson Product Coefficiency

$$r = \frac{\Sigma(X - X)(Y - Y)}{\sqrt{\Sigma(X - X)^2 \, \Sigma(Y - Y)^2}}$$

Note that the Pearson Product Coefficiency Correlation should be used only with interval/ratio data. You should not use this correlation with a nominal datum (e.g., sex) and correlate it with an interval/ratio datum (e.g., income). Other types of measures are used to correlate nominal data. What you should know is the purpose of a correlational study and what it means and doesn't mean.

Chi-square Analysis

Chi-square is the appropriate test of significance for nominal or ordinal data. Such tests that require only nominal or ordinal data are sometimes referred to as nonparametric tests (tests that use interval or ratio data are called parametric tests). For example, a chi-square analysis would be used to determine the difference between the voting practices of males and females on whether they tend to vote democratic or republican.

The chi-square was designed to be used with nominal data. Generally speaking, a chi-square is defined as the sum of the squared differences between the observed frequency and the expected frequency, divided by the expected frequency. Now this sounds like a mouthful, so here is a diagram of the formula:

$$x^2 = \sum \frac{(0 - E)^2}{E}$$

You can use a chi-square to determine (1) whether various groups or subgroups are similar; (2) whether there is a relationship between two variables; or (3) whether there is a significant difference between two proportions.

It is not the intent of this book to provide you with all of the gory details on how to compute a chi-square. Just remember that it is a good test to use in correlating nominal data.

Test of Means Analysis

This type of analysis is used with interval/ratio data to compare the means of two groups. For example, imagine that you are teaching two classes on vital statistics. In one class you decide to lecture, using this textbook as the mainstay of the course. In your other class, you decide that you want to do away with the lectures and the book and just give them handouts, with an occasional break to read poetry (your premise is that the more relaxed they are, the better they will learn vital statistics).

So throughout the semester you drill into your first class all of the formulas and theories in a intense series of lectures. In the other class, you put on a Hawaiian shirt and thongs and sit back and try to get the class to relax along with you. At the end of the semester you give them both the same final (the only item you are using to determine the student's grade). The lecture class scores on the average 75 (out of 100 possible). The "relaxed" class scores an average of 77. The SD of the first group is 6.5, and the SD of the second group is 6.6. Based on these results, did the "relaxed" approach do a better job at teaching vital statistics than the stand-up "lecture" version?

The relaxed class did score better, but was that difference due to the fact that they actually did learn more, or was it merely due to chance? This is where the test of means statistical analysis comes in. When one wants to compare the means of two groups, a *test of means*, or *t-test*, is the best approach. Again, you never need to do this by hand, but when you do a t-test you will get a *t* value. By looking this value (number) up in a special chart in any statistics text, you can determine whether or not this difference was due to chance or whether it was due to the intervention. (Most statistical software programs will give you both the *t* value and its probability.) In other words, you want to determine if this difference was significant.

Significance

This is another important concept in statistical analysis. To explain this term, let me give you an example. Let's say that I told you I had a magic coin, which tends to come up heads more often than tails. If this were true, I am sure that you would want to purchase this coin from me so that you could impress your friends and make money off of your enemies.

What would it take to convince you that this is a magic coin? If I flipped it one hundred times and it came up heads fifty-one times, would you consider this a magic coin? Probably not, but if you do, please give me a call. I've got a bunch of magic coins I'll sell you.

What if I flipped it one hundred times and it came up heads sixty times? Would that convince you? Just what would it take to convince you that this was a magic coin? Some might say that it would have to come up heads one hundred times; others may say that if it came up heads 90% of the time it would be considered magic.

Well, research is somewhat like a magic coin. A result occurs, and the researcher tries to determine if that result is due to some factor. If this researcher repeated his/her study one hundred times, how many times would he/she need to get the same results to convince you that this particular intervention is significant? That *level of significance* is up to the researcher and the consumer to determine. Typically, the researcher will set the level of significance prior to the study. This level can vary, but often in the behavioral sciences, the .05 level of significance is most common. What does .05 mean? It means that the researcher will not accept any findings unless there's less than a 5% chance that it was due to chance. The researcher is basically saying that he/she is 95% confident that the results of his/her study were due to a particular intervention. Anything above .05 is not acceptable—although for some researchers a level of significance at .10 would be acceptable.

Getting back to my coin. If I knew someone had a coin that would turn up heads 95% of the time, I'd probably hock my house to buy it. I'd be willing to take that 5% chance that when I bet other people, I would lose. In the long run, I'd win 95% of the time. And in research, there is hardly ever perfection or 100%.

Now let's go back to the two classes you taught. The relaxed class scored on the average 77, while the lecture class scored 75. If you would run a t-test, get the *t* value, and look it up in a special chart (available in any statistics text), it would tell you the probability that this was due to the intervention. If the probability was less than .05, then you may be willing to accept the difference in your teaching styles as significant. You may be able to conclude that the new teaching style did indeed improve the students' learning. If the probability was above .05, then you can probably state that the reason the relaxed class scored so well was due to chance and not the teaching strategy.

Keep in mind that you can never be 100% positive that your new teaching style is better. There could be a number of reasons why that class scored so well. One of the most logical reasons is that the students in your relaxed class were smarter to begin with. There's always a chance that you are wrong. Obviously, the stricter (or lower) the level of significance, the more positive or sure you can be.

To reiterate what was stated earlier, the level of significance is set by the researcher. What may be appropriate for one study may be totally inappropriate for another. For example, suppose you were to enter the hospital for a relatively simple hernia repair surgery. You would naturally be concerned and you would ask your surgeon what are your chances of complete recovery from the surgery. Your physician says that you have a 95% ch nce of surviving the surgery. Would you feel comfortable with that percentage? I don t know about you, but I would probably find another surgeon. Even 99% isn't good enough for me—at least not with simple surgery (I may accept those numbers if I were going to have a heart transplant). For the hernia operation, I would hope that the odds of making it out of surgery would be 100%, but since nothing is 100%, it would be nice if the o lds were better than 999 out of 1,000 that I would make it.

The t-test is the statistical approach to use when you want to determine whether there is a significant difference between two groups. Various factors can affect this significance. One of the most pronounced is the size of the groups. For example, let's say you had five students in your relaxed class compared to six students in your lecture class. A difference of three points (i.e., students in the relaxed group averaged 45 while the lecture students averaged 48) would mean nothing in this case. Now, imagine that the relaxed class had three hundred students and your lecture class also had three hundred students. There's a very good chance that a difference of two points would be a significant difference.

Analysis of Variance

Analysis of variance, or ANOVA, is the statistical test that is used when you have three or more groups that you want to compare. For example, in addition to the relaxed class and the lecture class, suppose you had a third class that was identical to the lecture class except that you sang the lecture notes (the "Cop Rock" of vital statistics). That group averaged 81 on their final. So now you need to compare the lecture group (score of 75), to the relaxed class (score of 77), to the singing class (score of 81). An ANOVA checks between each group and within each group to determine whether or not there is a significant difference. If there is a significance difference, the researcher has to do a post-hoc analysis to determine where the difference lies—was it between the 81 and 77, the 81 and 75, or the 77 and 75, or between more than one of the above comparisons. It's possible that singing to the class (score of 81) may be significantly more effective than lecturing (score of 75) or relaxing the class (score of 75), but there may be no difference between the lecture or relaxed groups.

3
Designing and Interpreting Tables and Graphs

Probably nothing sets a person apart as a true professional more than the ability to design good quality tables and graphs. Fortunately, computers are now able to do much of the tedious work. The vital statistician merely needs to punch the data into the program, and the system then transfers the information into the chosen table and/or graph. Programs such as Harvard Graphics, Microsoft Excel, and DrawPerfect are excellent for designing tables and graphs.

First, let's define terms. A *table* is an organized attempt to relay data/information to the reader in a simple and comprehensive format. The table consists of a title, headings, subheadings, categories, and data. A *graph* is a pictorial representation of data. The most common graphs are line graphs, histograms, bar graphs, and pie graphs. All graphs have some description of the results below them.

Tables

The key to producing a good table is to make it short, concise, and simple. Health educators who violate these principles tend to have their tables overlooked. It's a bias of mine that I would rather look at several tables than one with a lot of data. Admit it, when you've seen tables that are so complex, it becomes very easy just to overlook them. Tables can provide your results/information in an informative and practical fashion. Let's look at each of the components of a table.

Title. It's hard to believe that something so simple can be so difficult at times. Your title needs to be straight to the point, unlike a thesis or dissertation title, which is supposed to be both wordy, confusing, and authoritative sounding. The title on a table should be concise. For example, the following are some examples of titles of tables from the December 1990 issue of the *American Journal of Public Health*:

Hypertension Awareness, Treatment, and Control Status among Three Hispanic Subgroups (Pappas, et al.)

Prevalence of Clinical High Blood Pressure, by Race/Ethnicity and Age (Geronimus, et al.)

Type and Location of Facial Injuries Experienced (N = 212 individuals) (Thompson, et al.)

Let's design a table reporting HIV infection. Perhaps the title would read "Percentage of HIV Infection, by Sex and Race/Ethnicity."

Heading. This highlights a main variable under investigation. For example:

Percentage of HIV Infection, by Sex and Race/Ethnicity

	Male		Female
Whites	Nonwhites	Whites	Nonwhites

The title is the "Percentage of HIV Infection, by Sex and Race/Ethnicity." The headings are male and female. Also note that this particular table has subheadings, which are the white and nonwhites sections under each sex.

Percentage of HIV Infection, by Sex and Race/Ethnicity

Sex	Male		Female	
Race	Whites	Nonwhites	Whites	Nonwhites

In this example, note that we have added the categories sex and race on the side. These designations are not needed in all cases. Since this table is self-explanatory, it could do without such categories. However, if you wanted to include various age groups, then age would be placed where sex and race are currently located.

Note that the title stated that the table was showing the percentage of males and females (white and nonwhites) suffering from HIV. Because of that, it is not necessary for you to add the percent sign to numbers. The data can be listed as just numbers.

Percentage of HIV Infection, by Sex and Race/Ethnicity

	Male		Female
Whites	Nonwhites	Whites	Nonwhites
52.3	37.1	2.7	7.7°

° .2 race/ethnicity is unknown

Source: Data from the November 1990 *HIV/AIDS Surveillance* pamphlet

Obviously, the example given here is relatively simple, but the same premise exists for the more elaborate tables. The key is to make sure that people can understand what you are trying to say. Nothing will frustrate them more than if you present tables that only baffle them. And they may get the feeling that you are trying to disguise the data.

Graphs

Graphs attempt to provide the reader/viewer with data in an understandable and pictorial or "graphic" format (thus, the word *graph*). Graphs typically will have two axes. The variable under study is typically placed on the horizontal axis. This axis is also referred to as the x-axis or the abscissa. The vertical axis is referred to as the ordinate axis or, as I prefer, the y-axis. The y-axis will list the number of cases, the rates, the percentages, or whatever you are studying about the variable on the x-axis. The description of the study is placed below the graph.

Line Graph

The *line graph* (sometimes referred to as a frequency polygon) is commonly used. As the name depicts, it is a line that varies with the measured item. Let's suppose that you want to chart the age of the students in a class you are teaching. You're fortunate in that you only have ten students and their ages are closely bunched together. First, you identify the axes. The x- (horizontal) axis will designate the various ages. You can choose whatever interval you desire, but for this example we'll use a one-year interval. Also, since the youngest age we have in this class is eighteen, there's really no need to start at zero (the intersection of the x and y axes). There's a nifty technique to inform the reader that you are not starting at zero. On the x-axis, at the intersection of the x- and y-axes, place a double slash—//. This lets the reader know that you have "slashed" the age groups from zero to seventeen. Now, if you had someone at age twelve, you would only be able to slash from zero to twelve, and then continue the intervals throughout the graph.

Let's imagine that you have the following ages of students: three at eighteen, two at nineteen, one at twenty, zero at twenty-one, and four at twenty-two. How would you graph this? First place a dot *over each age group* at the appropriate number. You would place a dot that intersects the age 18 on the x-axis and the 3 on the y-axis. Place a dot over the 19 intersecting the 2 on the y-axis. Keep going for all five age groups. Look at figure 3.1 for assistance.

Once you have all the dots in place, you can then connect them with a straight line between each age group. For the first age group (18), you need to start your line at the intersection of the x and y axes. Note that you have no one at age 21, so your line would touch the x-axis line. Finally, after your age group of 22, you have one of two choices. Either end the line right there or add another age group of 23 and "anchor" the line at age 23. Of course, since you have no one that age, that anchor would be on the x-axis (as with the age 21 group). Note that there is a description of the information below the graph.

Histogram Graph

Using the same information as in figure 3.1, let's put it in a histogram. A *histogram* starts out the same way as the line graph. But after you place the dots corresponding to the numbers in each group, you add columns. Thus, for the eighteen-year-old group, you draw a column from the x-axis to the number 3 of the y-axis. The columns of each group should extend halfway between the age group identifier and the other age groups on both sides. Figure 3.2 demonstrates the histogram.

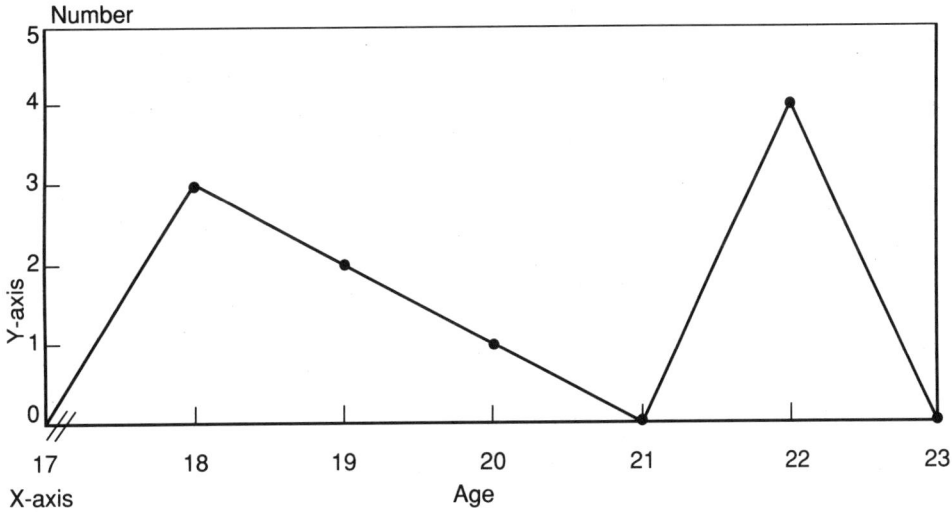

Age Breakdown of Students in Reader's Classroom

Fig. 3.1. Example of a line graph

Bar Graph

A bar graph is another popular graph used in the literature. The *bar graph* may at first appear to be the same as a histogram, but there are a couple of major differences. First, there's a space between each column, whereas the histogram has touching columns. The reason for this is the second major difference between a bar graph and a histogram. The variables under study on the x-axis in a histogram are continuous. Figure 3.2 shows that the ages represented on the x-axis are in logical order: 18 is before 19, 19 is before 20, etc. A histogram is used when you have a continuum on the x-axis. A bar graph is used when there is not a continuous variable.

For example, let's say you wanted to identify the various types of jobs that this class of yours has held. Ironically, every person has had only one job in one of the following four categories: gas station attendant, grocery store clerk, fast food server, salami maker. As you can tell from this grouping of jobs, each job stands by itself. One isn't contingent upon the other. Figure 3.3 demonstrates what this graph would look like. As you will note, the various jobs are listed on the x-axis, while the number of students who have had such a job is listed on the y-axis.

Two students have worked at gas stations; three have worked in grocery stores; one has worked in a fast food restaurant; and four have worked as salami makers. The columns on a bar graph can be narrower than those of a histogram, and typically, the edges of the bars do not touch.

The vital statistician can also depict several types of data on a line graph, histogram, and bar graph. For example, in figure 3.4 you will note that there are three lines on the graph. One line represents external causes, another line represents natural causes, and the third line represents all causes.

The following bar graph, figure 3.5, is an example of how a researcher has included both white and black athletes' injuries on the same graph.

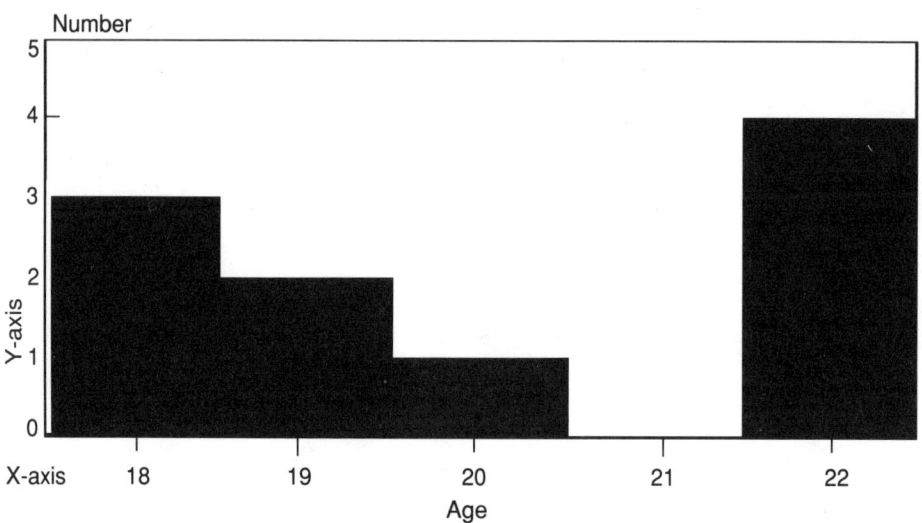

Age Breakdown of Students in Reader's Classroom

Fig. 3.2. Example of a histogram graph

Pie Graph

The final graph is the *pie graph*, which is a circular pictorial of the data. The "pie" is divided into various sections, typically a percentage of the total. Again, using the data from figure 3.1, the various percentages of each age group would be: age 18—30%; age 19—20%; age 20—10%; age 21—0%; and age 22—40%. The pie graph below indicates such a breakdown. If you have a computerized program to draw graphs, the pie chart can have an "exploding" pie, which means that a section of the pie is slightly removed from the rest of the pie. This is nice if you are highlighting a particular point in a paper. In addition, your pie can be a 3-D version, which not only shows the top but part of the side as well. The data from figure 3.1 are shown in pie graph format in figure 3.6.

Tables and graphs can be important tools in the vital statistician's job. It is important to communicate ideas effectively, and tables and graphs can help do that. Remember that both tables and graphs should be simple, concise, and to the point.

It's probably a good idea to review other textbooks that can give more specific information on compiling tables. If you are working on your thesis or dissertation, it's important for you to follow your particular graduate school guidelines. If you are using the APA format, it's probably a good idea to purchase the most current edition of the *Publication Manual of the American Psychological Association*.

Interpreting Tables

Besides having the ability to produce a good table or graph, the vital statistician needs to be able to interpret tables. For example, if you were presented the information in table 3.1, what would it mean to you?

When you look at this table, it should be clear that it gives no information on how

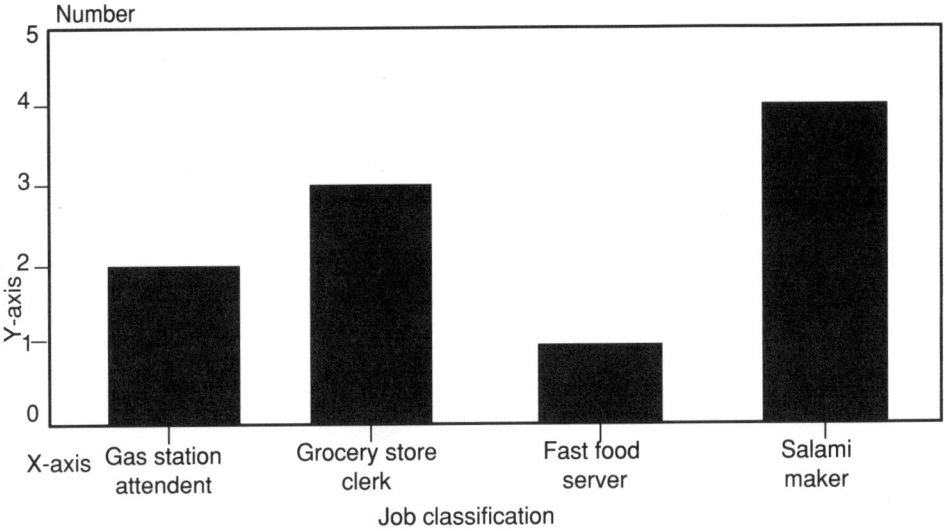

Type of Job Held by Students in the Reader's Classroom

Fig. 3.3. Example of a bar graph

the data were obtained. Were the reported cases of dingleitis reported through interviews, medical records, public health records, or what? In addition, one cannot be sure whether these "cases" are individuals or episodes (spells). In other words, if a person had dingleitis twice in one year, did he/she count as one or two cases?

All that one can state from the above data is that there is an increase of dingleitis between each of the reported years—you will note that the 1990 reported cases is three times that of the 1960 citation.

Another certainty that you can state is the overall extent of the increase. It can be reported in absolute or relative terms. The *absolute difference* is 1,600 cases (2,400 cases reported in 1990 minus 800 cases reported in 1960). The *relative difference*, as reported in the preceding paragraph, is a simple ratio: 2,400 ÷ 800 = 3.

The third point that you can be certain of is that the increase of dingleitis is not

**Table 3.1. Number of Cases of Acute Dingleitis
in Tokerville in Selected Years, 1960–1990**

Year	Cases
1960	800
1965	1,200
1970	1,600
1975	1,800
1980	2,000
1985	2,200
1990	2,400

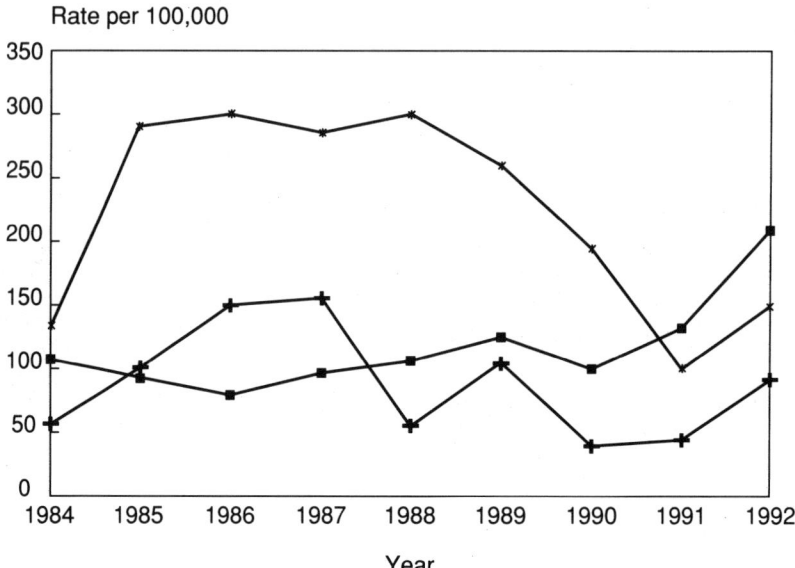

Mortality Rates of Female Inmates of the Rhode Island State Prison System,
from Natural, External, and All Causes

    ━■━ Natural causes   ━✛━ External causes   ━✳━ All causes

Fig. 3.4. Line graph depicting several types of data

consistent. In other words, in one five-year period dingleitis increased by 400 cases, whereas in another five-year period it increased by only 200 cases.

The vital statistician might hypothesize that the facts indicate sanitary conditions worsened, the population grew in size, or the number of deaths from dingleitis increased. These are not, however, empirical facts, but inferences. Inferences are acceptable, but vital statisticians must be able to differentiate between what they are certain of and what is being inferred. Basically, table 3.1 is poorly written, and it provides little information. Now look at table 3.2.

Table 3.2 shows the number of cases of dingleitis in Kittown and Sarvtown in 1985 and 1987. Health programs for preventing dingleitis were introduced in both towns in 1986. Let's calculate the absolute and relative changes in each town. The absolute difference in Kittown was −50 (50 −100), while the absolute difference in Sarvtown was

**Table 3.2. Number of Cases of Dingleitis
in Kittown and Sarvtown**

Year	Kittown	Sarvtown
1985	100	1,000
1987	50	8,000

Percent of injuries

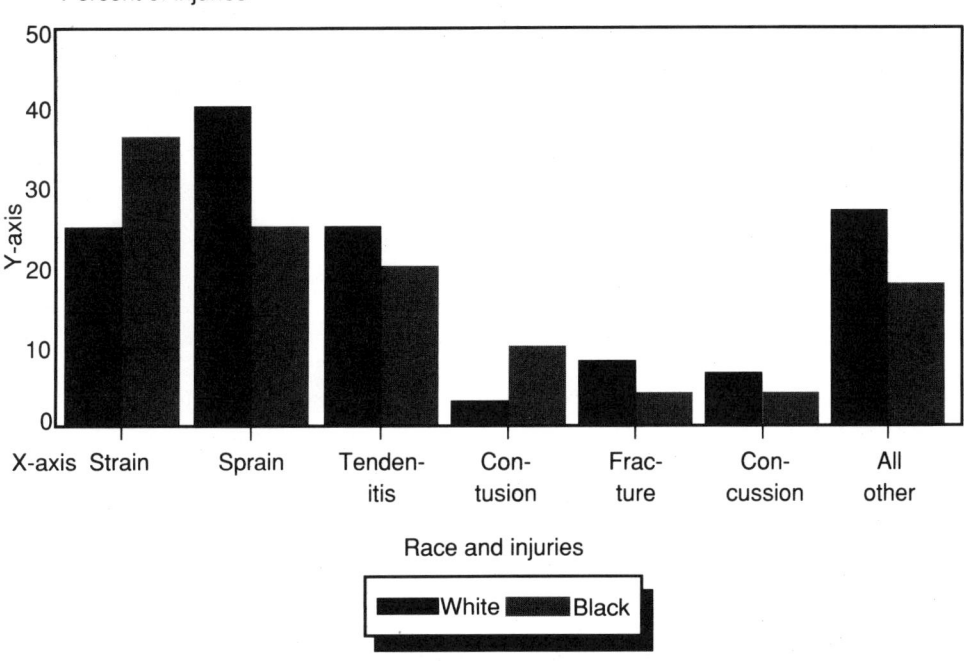

Race and injuries

Percent of Injuries by Type among White and Black Athletes
in Matched Sports at a Large University

Fig. 3.5. Bar graph depicting several types of data

7,000 (8,000 − 1,000). The relative difference in Kittown was a one-half *reduction* (50 ÷ 100). The relative difference in Sarvtown was an *increase* of eight times (8,000 ÷ 1,000).

In which town is there stronger evidence that the program was effective in reducing the occurrence of dingleitis? From the table, it looks like Kittown has seen a rather dramatic drop in the reported cases of dingleitis. But one cannot be sure because of unknown factors such as population growth or age distribution (perhaps only young children get dingleitis and maybe Kittown has become a retirement community). Ideally, the table should have listed the populations of both towns.

Here are two more examples to work on.

Suppose you are a health administrator concerned with the provision of facilities for health care in these towns. Table 3.3 shows the numbers of new patients with end-

**Table 3.3. Number of Patients Requiring Dialysis
in Kittown and Sarvtown**

Year	Kittown	Sarvtown
1992	30	2,000
1994	90	3,000

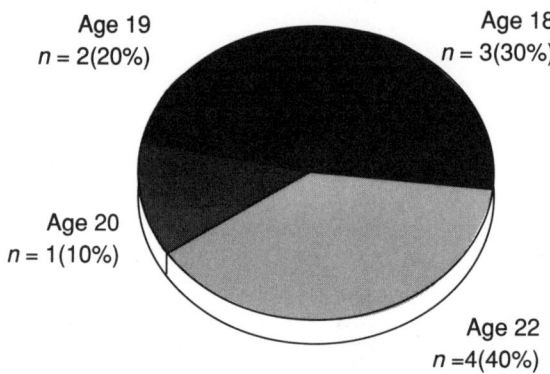

Age Breakdown of Students in the Reader's Classroom

Fig. 3.6. Example of a pie graph

stage dingleitis, which requires dialysis (a life-saving, but elaborate and expensive form of treatment), in two regions in 1992 and 1994. Calculate the absolute and relative changes. Looking forward to 1995, in which region would the increase concern you more? You see that there was a 3-fold increase in Kittown, whereas there was a 1.5-fold increase in Sarvtown. Yet Sarvtown has seen many more people requiring dialysis than Kittown. Sometimes absolute numbers can play a more important factor than the relative difference, whereas at other times the relative difference is more appropriate than the absolute number.

Table 3.4 shows the number of infant deaths in the same two regions in 1992 and 1994; the numbers of births did not change. Programs aimed at reducing infant mortality were started in both regions in 1986.

1. In which region is there more convincing evidence that the reduction in mortality was caused by the program?
2. If the program can be continued in only one region, which would you choose? (Assume that the reductions are caused by the program.)

There are a number of ways to answer question one. There was a fivefold decrease in Kittown, yet proponents for Sarvtown would argue that although there was only a reduction of 1.25-fold, there were more individuals (1,000 compared to only 240).

For question two, one must take into account a number of factors, but the bottom line comes down to whether the decision makers are more apt to be convinced by raw

Table 3.4. Number of Infant Deaths in Kittown and Sarvtown

Year	Kittown	Sarvtown
1992	300	5,000
1994	60	4,000

**Table 3.5. Total Deaths Registered—U.S. Death Registration,
Selected States for Selected Years**

Year	Deaths (in thousands)
1910	686
1930	2,236
1950	2,834
1970	3,422
1990	2,842

numbers or by a proportional reduction (in other words, what sounds better: a reduction by 1,000 individuals, or a fivefold reduction).

Looking at the data in table 3.5 and using death as an indicator, do you think that Americans of 1990 are less healthy than their predecessors? What makes you think that?

A few points to ponder about table 3.5:

1. These are data for the United States and only for death registration states. Hence, prior to 1933 they do not refer to the whole nation, because all states were not yet included in the death registration system.
2. The data are for selected years. Showing years ending in zero is common in tables containing health information, because these are the years of the decennial U.S. Census of Population and Housing.
3. The figures given are numbers of deaths registered.
4. These figures appear to be small because they are in thousands.

4

Ratio, Proportion, Percentage, and Rate

Part of the reason for the collection of vital statistics is to help the public health official make decisions regarding the planning and/or implementing of various institutional programs. Yet numbers can be confusing and even misrepresented. By now we are all aware of that age-old saying, "There are lies, damned lies, and statistics." There is no doubt that the use of statistics by unethical individuals can bend the truth. Yet omission, instead of commission, can be just as confusing and perhaps even as unethical.

One should keep in mind the importance of vital statistics in the planning of programs. Rarely will a county, state, or region be assessed only by vital statistics data before any major project is approved or denied. Yet in many instances, vital statistics will allow a community the opportunity to present its case. An example might be helpful: In August of 1990, the Centers for Disease Control (CDC) (now the Centers for Disease Control and Prevention) announced a Request for Proposals (RFPs) to coordinate HIV education for college students. Although any state could apply, the CDC announced that only five would be funded from those states with the highest rates of AIDS cases. Those ten states were New York, Illinois, New Jersey, Puerto Rico, Florida, Texas, Pennsylvania, California, Massachusetts, and Georgia. The other forty states were ineligible. Why? Because the CDC decided that only those states with sufficiently high numbers of AIDS cases were eligible. How did they determine these states? They looked at their vital statistics.

Many individuals may feel that this is unfair and maybe that a program in Minnesota could have been the best proposal in the country. But it didn't matter, because Minnesota wasn't eligible for the funding. The point that I am trying to make is that whether it is fair or unfair, decisions are often made based on available vital statistics. Yet because many decisions are made based on this approach, the statistics can often be misused, abused, or misrepresented. As public health educators, it is imperative that you learn to fight fire with fire and to know when people are trying to bluff you.

Vital statistics are typically computed by several types of processes for data analysis. The simplest, ratio, will be discussed first, then proportion, percentage, and, briefly, rate. Since rate is most commonly used to impart information, the next chapter is devoted exclusively to this process of data analysis.

Ratio

Ratio is a pretty simple process used to measure data. Basically, you divide the population that you are studying into two parts. The ratio is stated as "so many cases of A to one case of B."

For example, suppose you wanted to identify the ratio of males to females in a particular county. The county states that there are ten thousand residents living within its boundaries. Of this number, six thousand are males and the remaining are females. To get the ratio of males to females in this community, simply divide the total of the males by the total of the females. It would look like the following:

$$\frac{6,000 \text{ (males)}}{4,000 \text{ (females)}} = 1.50 \text{ (ratio of males to females)}$$

So, in this particular community, there are 1.50 males for every 1.00 female. Or you can state that for every 1.00 female, there are 1.50 males. Or you could multiply each by a constant (such as 10) and then state that there are 15 males for every 10 females in this county.

It really doesn't matter which number is the numerator (the one above the line), but many people prefer the larger of the two numbers as the numerator so that you end up with a whole number compared to a smaller number. But, if we swapped the numbers, it would look like this:

$$\frac{4,000 \text{ (females)}}{6,000 \text{ (males)}} = .67 \text{ (ratio of females to males)}$$

So, using this formula, you could say that for every .67 females in your county, there is 1.00 male. Or, for every 1.00 male, there are .67 females. As you can see, the concept is the same, but it doesn't really make much sense. Of course, if you multiply each by a constant of 100, then you could say that for every 67 females, there are 100 males, which conceptually makes a little more sense.

The idea of a ratio is to give the vital statistician a simple comparison. A ratio could compare the number of nonmarital births (or in some states they are called illegitimate births) to those births of married women. You could also figure a ratio of the number of auto fatalities to the total of all other accident fatalities. You could figure an age-specific death rate for both males and females (to be discussed in chapter 5) and then do a ratio comparison between the two. For example, if the death rate of eighteen-year-old males is ten per thousand (10/1,000) and the death rate of eighteen-year-old females is 5/1,000, you could do a ratio that would show that for every 1 eighteen-year-old female that dies, 2 eighteen-year-old males die. The formula would be:

$$\frac{10 \text{ (males per thousand)}}{5 \text{ (females per thousand)}} = 2 \text{ (ratio of males to females)}$$

If you use a ratio, you must split the population you are studying into two parts, and

Table 4.1. Proportional Distribution of Causes of Death

Cause of Death	No. of Cases	Proportion
Heart disease	250	
Cancer	150	
Accidents	100	
Chronic obstructed pulmonary disease	60	
Flu/pneumonia	50	
Diabetes	50	
Other	140	
Total deaths	800	1.00

you must use the same measurement (for example births). Also, the data in both the numerator and the denominator should be collected during the same time period. It probably wouldn't make sense to figure a ratio of births in 1991 to those in 1971. In addition, it probably wouldn't make sense to compare the number of people dying of heart disease to the number of people suffering from epilepsy.

Proportion

Proportion is another process used in analyzing data. A *proportion* relates the comparison in a decimal statement. Referring to our earlier example, in a county of ten thousand, there are six thousand males and four thousand females. What proportion of the population is male? To figure this out, you need to divide the specific subject (in this case males) by the total population (remember with the ratio you just divided males by females—in this case you'll be dividing 6,000 males by the total population of 10,000 [4,000 females + 6,000 males]). Thus, to get the proportion of males in this particular county, the following formula is needed:

$$\text{Proportion of males} = \frac{6,000 \text{ (males)}}{10,000 \text{ (males + females)}} = .60$$

Thus, the proportion of males in this county is .60. If you wanted to determine the proportion of females in this county, you would put the 4,000 females above the line and divide by 10,000 (the total population). The proportion is .40. It's important to note that when you add up all of the various proportions, they should total 1.00. If they total less, or more, you've done something wrong.

Proportion Practice Problem

Table 4.1 relates the causes of death in a particular community. Determine the proportion that each cause of death plays in this community. In this particular example, do not round off. Usually, rounding off to the nearest hundredth is acceptable. In some

Table 4.1A. Proportional Distribution of Causes of Death—Answers

Cause of Death	No. of Cases	Proportion
Heart disease	250	.3125
Cancer	150	.1875
Accidents	100	.1250
Chronic obstructed pulmonary disease	60	.0750
Flu/pneumonia	50	.0625
Diabetes	50	.0625
Other	140	.1750
Total deaths	800	1.0000

instances, rounding off to the nearest tenth is acceptable as well. The answers can be found in table 4.1A.

Percentage

A *percentage* is simply a proportion that is multiplied by 100 and given a percent sign. Thus, in table 4.1A, the proportion of individuals dying from heart disease is .3125. If we multiply that number by 100, it would then be 31.25%. It means the same as .3125, but it's another way of expressing data. Again, it depends on the population you are trying to reach. Some may feel more comfortable with proportions, and others may feel more comfortable with percentages.

Rate

A rate is perhaps the most common process of statistical analysis in vital statistics. It is so important that the next chapter is devoted entirely to this process.

Practice Problems

Answers can be found at the end of this chapter.

Practice Problem One

There are 1,000 reported cases of computeritis in Software County. The county's population is 25,000, of which 13,000 are males and 12,000 are females. Of the 1,000 cases of computeritis, 750 involved males.

1. What is the proportion of males in Software County? What is the ratio of males to females?

Table 4.2. Proportional Distribution of Causes of Death, by Age Group

Age Group	No. of Cases	Population
0–9	12	6,800
10–19	41	8,400
20–29	62	5,600
30–39	71	5,200
40+	55	14,000
Total	241	40,000

2. What is the proportion of males who suffer computeritis? What is the ratio of males to females who suffer computeritis?

3. What is the proportion of males who do not suffer computeritis? What is the ratio of males to females who do not suffer computeritis?

During 1988, a total of 241 cases of computeritis were reported from a community having a population of 40,000. Of the 241 cases of computeritis, 44 occurred during the period of January through March; 61 occurred during the period of April through June; none during July through September; and 136 during October through December. Further investigation of the 241 cases of computeritis revealed that 76 cases involved males and the rest females. The number of males in the community was 18,500.

4. Calculate the proportional distribution of the cases by season.

5. Determine the ratio of male cases to female cases.

6. Calculate the proportional distribution of the cases by sex.

Another item of information obtained during the investigation was the age of the person who had the disease. This information was tabulated by age group and is presented in table 4.2. Also given is the total number of people in each of these age groups who lived in the community.

7. Calculate the proportional distribution of the cases by age.

Practice Problem Two

During 1986, a total of 126 cases of the St. Louis Drip (SLD), an irritating runny nose, was reported from a community having a population of 20,000. Of the 126 cases of SLD previously referred to, 0 occurred during the period of January through March; 5 occurred during the period of April through June; 113 occurred during July through September; and 8 occurred during October through December.

8. Calculate the proportional distribution of the cases by season.

Table 4.3. Cases of SLD, by Age Group

Age Group	No. of Cases	Population
0–9	17	3,400
10–19	18	4,200
20–29	9	2,800
30–39	11	2,600
40+	71	7,000
Total	126	20,000

Further investigation of the 126 cases of SLD revealed that 67 cases involved males and the rest females. The number of males in the community was 9,200.

9. Determine the ratio of male cases to female cases.

10. Calculate the proportional distribution of the cases by sex.

Another item of information obtained during the investigation was the age of the person who had the disease. This information was tabulated by age group and is presented in table 4.3. Also given is the total number of people in each of these age groups who lived in the community.

11. Calculate the proportional distribution of the cases by age.

Practice Problem Three

During 1988, a total of 666 cases of dingleitis were reported from a community having a population of 30,000. Dingleitis is a dreaded disease that involves the inflammation of one's dingle. Of the 666 cases of dingleitis, 218 occurred during the period of January through March; 61 occurred during the period of April through June; 255 during July through September; and 132 during October through December.

12. Calculate the proportional distribution of the cases by season.

Further investigation of 666 cases of dingleitis revealed that 476 cases involved males and the rest females. The number of males in the community was 14,200.

13. Calculate the proportional distribution of the cases by sex.

Another item of information obtained during the investigation was the age of the person who had the disease. This information was tabulated by age group and is presented in table 4.4. Also given is the total number of people in each of these age groups who lived in the community.

14. Calculate the proportional distribution of the cases by age.

Table 4.4. Cases of Dingleitis, by Age Group

Age Group	No. of Cases	Population
0–9	100	7,800
10–19	99	6,500
20–29	65	7,600
30–39	159	4,200
40+	243	3,900
Total	666	30,000

Answers to Practice Problems

1. The proportion of males in Software County is .52. The formula for this is 13,000/25,000.

   The ratio of males to females is 1.08 to 1.00. The formula for this is 13,000/12,000.

2. The proportion of males who suffer from computeritis is .75. You determine this by the following formula: 750/1,000. There are 750 males who suffer from computeritis, and 250 females who suffer from the same affliction. To determine the ratio of males to females, you would use the following formula: 750/250. The answer is 3.00 to 1.00.

3. The proportion of noninfected males is determined by dividing the number of noninfected males by the total number of noninfected individuals. You determine that by first listing those individuals who do not suffer computeritis. Among the 13,000 males in Software County, 12,250 are noninfected; among the 12,000 females, 11,750 are noninfected. 12,250 (males)/24,000 (total of noninfected individuals) = .51.

   There are 12,250 males not suffering from computeritis, and 11,750 females. Thus, a ratio of males to females not suffering from this disease is determined by the formula 12,250/11,750. The answer is 1.04 males to 1.00 female.

4. For January through March, the proportion is .18 (44/241); for April through June, .25 (61/241); for July through September, 0 (0/241); for October through December .56 (136/241).

5. There were 76 males and 165 females suffering from computeritis. To get a ratio of male cases to female cases you do the following: 76/165. The answer is .46 male to 1.00 female.

6. To figure the proportion by sex, divide the number of infected males and females each by the number of the total infected population. For males, 76/241 reveals a proportion of .31; for females, 165/241 reveals a proportion of .68 (note that I am rounding off to the nearest hundredth).

7. For the 0–9 age group, 12/241 = .04; for 10–19, 41/241 = .17; for 20–29, 62/241 = .26; for 30–39, 71/241 = .29; for 40+, 55/241 = .23. Note that the population is unrelated to this problem.

8. For January through March, the proportion is 0 (0/126); for April through June, .04 (5/126); for July through September, .90 (113/126); for October through December, .06 (8/126).

9. There were 67 males suffering from SLD and 59 females. The formula is 67/59. The answer is 1.14 males to 1.00 female.

10. Of the 126 cases, 67 were males and 59 were females. To find the proportion of males, 67/126 = .53. For females, 59/126 = .47.

11. For the 0–9 age group 17/126 = .13; for 10–19, 18/126 = .14; for 20–29, 9/126 = .07; for 30–39, 11/126 = .09; for 40+, 71/126 = .56.

12. For January through March the proportion is .33 (218/666); for April through June, .09 (61/666); for July through September, .38 (255/666); for October through December, .20 (132/666).

13. Of the 666 cases, 476 were males and 190 were females. To find the proportion of males, 476/666 = .71; for females, 190/666 = .29.

14. For the 0–9 age group, 100/666 = .15; for 10–19, 99/666 = .149; for 20–29, 65/666 = .098; for 30–39, 159/666 = .239; for the 40+, 243/666 = .365.

5

Rate

As indicated in chapter 4, rate is probably the most common process used to analyze and report vital statistics. In almost all cases, government documents provide information based on rates. When used properly, this process can provide invaluable information on the status of health in a county, state, or country. In this chapter I discuss rate types and how to obtain specific rates.

Note the following statistics computed from two communities.

Deaths Due to Dingleitis, 1991

Smithville	Clarksburg
20,000	2,000

Based on this information, what would be your first impression? It's quite clear that Smithville has ten times the number of reported deaths due to dingleitis during 1991. But what else can you say from the results? There's nothing of certainty other than that Smithville has more reported dingleitis deaths than Clarksburg during 1991 and that a total of 22,000 deaths from dingleitis was identified during that year. Anything else you might say is merely conjecture or an educated guess.

Part of the difficulty of reporting information is analyzing what is included in the table or graph. Now, if I were to say that the total population of Smithville is 2,000,000 and that the total population of Clarksburg is 20,000, what would that tell you? Even before doing any statistical analysis on such information, it appears that Clarksburg has a higher proportion of deaths from dingleitis.

This is where various rate processes are most often used. A *rate* is a method of describing the occurrence of a particular disease (or death) in relatively simple terms. People have difficulty thinking in large numbers, such as a billion. For that matter, many people have difficulty conceptualizing a million. In addition, people often have difficulty grasping decimals. We are comfortable with the use of decimals in money—seventy-five cents is reported as .75. Yet when we say that a gallon of gas costs $1.599, it seems strange. But it's the same as saying that gas costs $1.59 and 9/10. (Why do the oil companies set their prices like that? The answer goes beyond the scope of this book, and

I don't want to violate any classified government secrets, but I believe it's related to perceived human gullibility.)

Rate Definition

A rate is a process of statistical analysis. The way to determine a rate for the above example is to first divide the number of people who died from dingleitis by the total number of the population. Thus, for Smithville, 20,000 individuals who died from dingleitis infection during 1991 is divided by a total population of 2,000,000, which gives you .01. (If you remember from your reading of the last chapter, this is a proportion.)

What does this mean? It's read one one-hundredth. This is where the use of a *base* comes in. A rate uses a base, whereas proportion uses the decimal number. There is no right or wrong base; it is used merely for classification. Thus, instead of saying that one-one-hundredth of the population in Smithville died from dingleitis during 1991, you could multiple .01 by 1,000. The result would then state that the number of people who died of dingleitis during 1991 was ten per one thousand (10/1,000).

Why did I choose 1,000? There's no particular reason, but being author of this book does give me special privileges. In spite of this, there was a method in my madness. I always try to choose a base that provides at least one whole number. For example, if I were to multiple .01 by 10,000, it would read 100/10,000—another acceptable figure. If I wanted to use a base of 100,000, the rate would be 1,000/100,000. Yet if I were to multiply the .01 by 10, it would read .10/100. I believe that says that for every one hundred people in Smithville, one-tenth of a person died. I don't know about you, but I find that very hard to visualize. Keep in mind that in many instances you are going to be reporting your results to a group of people who are not as competent in the interpretation of vital statistics. Thus, I would suggest that you keep it simple. The key in choosing a base is to make sure that you use it consistently with the compared data. For example, don't use a base of 1,000 for Smithville and a base of 10,000 for Clarksburg. It muddies the waters and makes comparisons difficult. Also keep in mind that .10/100, 1/1,000, 10/10,000, and 100/100,000 all mean the same: the rate is identical.

Let's figure another example. Clarksburg has a total of 2,000 individuals out of a population of 20,000 who died from dingleitis in 1991. First, divide the number of cases by the population. The number you get on your calculator should be .10. Following the same format as earlier, multiply that .10 by a base of 1,000. The reading should be 100/1,000, or for every 1,000 residents in Clarksburg, 100 died from dingleitis during 1991.

Now let's compare the rate of dingleitis infection in Smithville to Clarksburg. For every 1,000 residents in Smithville, 10 became infected with dingleitis. In Clarksburg, for every 1,000 residents, 100 became infected. By looking at this data, it is quite clear that Clarksburg has a much higher rate of dingleitis death than Smithville. In fact, that rate is ten times higher.

What do you think accounts for this difference? You can conjecture; you can give an educated guess; but you don't really know. You could look at other demographic data to ascertain some of these reasons. The point I am trying to make is that even among the best vital statisticians, there is a certain amount of guesswork as to the reasons why. It is important that we are aware that guesswork does take place. We also need to know when those individuals are giving their *educated guesses*. All too often, we hear "experts" citing specific rates and then they cite the reasons. Unless they have other sources of vital statistics or other demographic information, all of those reasons are just guesswork. You can't discount these educated guesses, but just keep them in the proper perspective.

Rate can be determined by the following formula:

$$\frac{\text{number of cases of } x}{\text{population at risk to } x} \times \text{base}$$

Rate is probably the most common statistical analysis that public health officials use in reporting vital statistics. It is the groundwork of all future work, so if you are confused at this point, I would suggest that you reread this section, and if you are still confused, give your instructor a call or visit. I know there are many individuals reading this book who are paranoid about anything to do with statistics. But I want to stress that understanding the rate process is very important and needs your undivided attention.

Rate Types

There are different rate types. The most basic is the *crude rate*, which is the number of individual cases being studied divided by the total number of the population. Now at first that seems sufficient, yet there are times when the crude rate is really inappropriate. For example, if a community of 10,000 had 100 births, what is the crude birthrate (use a base of 1,000). For every 1,000 residents in this community, 10 gave birth. Another way of saying this is that the crude birth rate is 10/1,000 (ten per thousand). Imagine that this same community of 10,000 had 50 deaths. What would be the crude death rate (using 1,000 as a base)? For every 1,000 residents, 5 died, so the crude death rate is 5/1,000.

Yet both of these rates could be more specific. For example, the crude birthrate takes into account a large portion of the population who cannot give birth (males). If one wanted to get a better idea on the rate of females giving birth, one could "fractionalize" the data into segments. In many circles of vital statistics, this is often referred to as the *fertility rate*, which is the number of women between the ages of 15 and 44 who give birth.

In a related comparison, age would certainly be an interesting factor. Of those one hundred births, what were the ages of the mothers? For example, if 10 of those births were to mothers between the ages of 15 and 18 and there were a total of 500 females in this age bracket, one could use that information to report an age-specific birthrate. In this case, the total number of births in the particular age group (10) would be divided by the total number of females in that age group (500). Thus, 10 divided by 500 times a base of 1,000 would give you the rate of births for this age bracket. The answer is 20/1,000. What that says is that for every 1,000 females in this community between the ages of 15 and 18, 20 will deliver a live birth. That in and of itself may not tell you a lot, but if you figure this for each age group, certain patterns may emerge.

Rate Practice Problem

Finish the rest of table 5.1. The answers follow in table 5.1A.

Table 5.1. Birthrates among Women of Selected Age Categories

Age Group	No. of Women	No. of Births	Birthrate°
15–18	500	10	
19–24	1,000	40	
25–34	2,500	30	
35–44	1,000	20	

°Rate per 1,000

Now, one could look at the table and say, "Hey, there aren't 1,000 females in the 15 to 18 age category in this community!" You're right, but the point of using rates (in this case the age-specific birthrate) is to describe the community in such a way that people can best understand it. When you are attempting to compare two or more communities, it is important to make sure that you are comparing apples to apples and not apples to oranges. So even if you indicate that the age-specific birthrate of women 15–18 is 20 births per 1,000 females (and the fact is that there are only 500 females), you are giving a general description of the community using equal measurements.

So anytime you break the rates into any specific grouping, such as age, sex, or even race, you are getting a *specific rate*. The above is an example of an age-specific birthrate (although technically you could say that it's also a sex-age-specific birthrate since it included only females, or it could be called an age-specific fertility rate). Later on in this text, you'll be able to give a age-race-sex-specific death rate. It will sound impressive, and your parents, spouses, and children will be proud of you, but really, it's not that difficult (but don't let them know this). The examples of the dingleitis death rates from the earlier example could be referred to as a disease-specific death rate, since the study looked specifically at those who died from dingleitis in 1991.

Other types of rates include incidence and prevalence. *Prevalence* is the total number of cases that exist (old and new). *Incidence* is the number of *new* cases during a certain time period.

Reported Flu Cases During 1991

Smithville	Clarksburg
4,000	400

These data show the total number of reported flu cases during 1991. In Smithville, 4,000 new cases of flu were reported in 1991, while Clarksburg saw 400 new cases during 1991. Since the data show the number of *new* cases of flu during 1991, this number is used to figure the incidence rate. Remembering that Smithville has a population of 2,000,000 and Clarksburg has a population of 20,000, the incidence rates for Smithville and Clarksburg are 2/1,000 and 20/1,000 respectively. Incidence is often used for those illnesses that are prominent during certain times of the year.

Let's add a new twist to this. Let's focus on the incidence rate of a fictitious disease entitled racheli. Once you acquire racheli you will always have it. You can reduce the discomfort from this disease, but eventually you will succumb to the disease. So instead

Table 5.1A. Birthrates among Women of Selected Age Categories—Answers

Age Group	No. of Women	No. of Births	Birthrate°
15–18	500	10	20
19–24	1,000	40	40
25–34	2,500	30	12
35–44	1,000	20	20

°Rate per 1,000

of the flu, let's focus on the incidence rate of reported racheli cases during 1991. You would need to look at the public health records to find the number of individuals who were diagnosed with racheli during 1991 and divide by the number of those individuals who are at risk of becoming infected. This last phase needs clarification. You would not add into that denominator those individuals who already have been diagnosed with racheli. So anyone who is reported as having racheli is out of the denominator equation.

Okay, look at the data below carefully. You will note the number of racheli cases reported during 1991 (first list), and the total number of cases at the end of 1991 (second list).

Reported Racheli Cases During 1991

Smithville	Clarksburg
4,000	400

Total Number of Reported Racheli Cases at End of 1991

Smithville	Clarksburg
20,000	2,000

To determine the incidence rate of racheli cases in 1991, you first need to determine the number of cases (4,000 and 400 respectively). Now, you need to determine the number of individuals who are vulnerable to developing racheli by looking at the reported cases in 1990. At the end of 1990, how many people lived in Smithville who did not have a reported case of racheli? First, before 1991, there were 16,000 reported cases of racheli (20,000 − 4,000)—thus, 2,000,000 (total population) minus 16,000 is equal to 1,984,000 individuals in Smithville who were not reported to have racheli at the end of 1990—the population at risk. The incidence rate for 1991 would be 4,000 divided by 1,984,000, times your base. Thus:

$$\frac{4,000 \text{ (no. of cases)}}{1,984,000 \text{ (population at risk)}} \times 1,000 = 2.0161/1,000$$

The incidence rate in 1991 of racheli in Smithville was 2.02 per 1,000 population. Does that make sense? If not, reread this section and/or ask your instructor for help.

The incidence rate during 1991 for racheli in Clarksburg would be determined in the same fashion. First, decide how many people were not infected at the end of 1990. You do this by first subtracting the number of cases in 1991 (400) from the total number of cases at the end of 1991 (2,000), which is equal to 1,600, the number of cases before 1991. The total population of Clarksburg was 20,000, so subtract 1,600 from 20,000, which equals 18,400. This gives you the number of individuals who were not reported to have a racheli case at the end of 1990—the population at risk. To determine the incidence rate, divide 400 by 18,400, multiply by a base of 1,000, and the rate should be 21.74 per 1,000. That states that during 1991, the rate of having an racheli case reported was 21.74 per 1,000 population.

So, to summarize how to determine the incidence rate, you need to do the following:

1. Determine the time period that you want to assess (in the above example, we chose the year 1991).
2. Determine the number of cases during that time period (in the above example we found that Smithville had 4,000 cases of racheli, while Clarksburg had 400 cases).
3. Determine the population at risk. Here you have to do a little math. In the example, we saw that 20,000 Smithville residents had racheli, with 4,000 of them reported during 1991; thus the population at risk was 2,000,000 minus 16,000 for a total of 1,984,000. In Clarksburg, 18,400 were at risk to develop racheli during 1991.
4. Divide the number of individuals developing the disease during your time slot (1991) by the population at risk and multiply by a base.

As you can see, this process involves a tremendous amount of work, and in most chronic diseases (or those diseases that once you have the disease, you always have it), it is much easier to compare in terms of prevalence (old and new cases).

Finally, the last type of rate you should be familiar with is the *standardized rate*. This type of rate is used primarily to compare two communities that have vastly different demographics. For example, how could someone compare the death rates between the state of Massachusetts and that of Florida? Massachusetts has an incredibly young population, and Florida is a state with a large senior population. Standardization allows a public health official to manipulate the vital statistics and make comparisons. This approach will be covered in chapter 6.

As discussed in chapter 4, ratio is a popular measurement and can be a means of simplifying numbers: for example, the ratio of males to females or the ratio of male cases of a particular disease to female cases of the same disease. Let's say that 100 males suffer from a particular disease and 50 females suffer from the same disease. You could figure a ratio and determine that for every 1 female, 2 males suffer from this particular disease. In this case, we are using *raw figures*—in other words, the actual number of people who are suffering from this ailment. As discussed earlier, there are drawbacks to using only raw numbers, and it would be more helpful if you could determine the rate of males and females who are suffering from the disease. In this same community where 100 males are suffering from this disease, let's say that there are 10,000 males. The rate computes to 10 per 1,000 males suffering from this disease. Let's also say that there are

9,000 females in this community (remember, 50 suffering from this disease). The rate would be 5.60 per 1,000 females suffering from this disease. Now the two rates, 10 for males and 5.60 for females, can be put into a ratio. 10 (males)/5.60 (females) = 1.79 males to every 1.00 female. The ratio of the male rate to the female rate is 1.79 males to every 1.00 female.

Practice Problems

Answers can be found at the end of this chapter.

Practice Problem One

Referring to the previous chapter on computeritis, remember that during 1988 a total of 241 cases of computeritis were reported from a community having a population of 40,000.

1. Calculate the rate of computeritis in the community during 1988.

Of the 241 cases of computeritis, 44 occurred during the period of January through March; 61 occurred during the period of April through June; none during July through September; and 136 during October through December.

2. Calculate the rates per 10,000 population for computeritis for each of the quarterly periods.

Further investigation of the 241 cases of computeritis revealed that 76 cases involved males and the rest females. The number of males in the community was 18,500.

3. Calculate the sex-specific disease rates per 10,000 population.

4. Using the rates figured in question 3, now determine the ratio of male cases to female cases and the ratio of male rate to the female rate.

Another item of information obtained during the investigation was the age of the person who had the disease. This information was tabulated by age group and is presented in table 5.2. Also given is the total number of people in each of these age groups who lived in the community.

5. Calculate the age-specific disease rates per 1,000 population for each of the age groups shown above.

Fifteen of the 241 cases died. Six were less than 7 years old and 9 were over 50 years old. Eight were females and 7 were males.

6. Calculate the following mortality rates per 100,000 population:

6a. community-wide mortality rate;

Table 5.2. Cases of Computeritis, by Age Group

Age Group	No. of Cases	Population
0–9	12	6,800
10–19	41	8,400
20–29	62	5,600
30–39	71	5,200
40+	55	14,000
Total	241	40,000

6b. age-specific mortality rate for the affected age groups;

6c. sex-specific mortality rates.

Practice Problem Two

During 1986, a total of 126 cases of the St. Louis Drip (SLD) was reported from a community having a population of 20,000.

7. Calculate the rate of SLD in the community during 1986.

Of the 126 cases of SLD previously referred to, none occurred during the period of January through March; 5 occurred during the period of April through June; 113 occurred during July through September; and 8 occurred during October through December.

8. Calculate the rates per 10,000 population for SLD for each of the quarterly periods.

Further investigation of the 126 cases of SLD revealed that 67 cases involved males and the rest females. The number of males in the community was 9,200.

9. Calculate the sex-specific disease rates per 10,000 population.

10. Using the rates figured in question 9, determine the ratio of male cases to female cases and the ratio of the male rate to the female rate.

Another item of information obtained during the investigation was the age of the person who had the disease. This information was tabulated by age group and is presented in table 5.3. Also given is the total number of people in each of these age groups who lived in the community.

11. Calculate the age-specific disease rates per 1,000 population for each of the age groups shown above.

Table 5.3. Cases of SLD, by Age Group

Age Group	No. of Cases	Population
0–9	17	3,400
10–19	18	4,200
20–29	9	2,800
30–39	11	2,600
40+	71	7,000
Total	126	20,000

Four of the 126 cases died. One was less than 9 years old and 3 were over 40 years of age. Two were males and 2 were females.

12. Calculate the following mortality rates per 100,000 population:

12a. community-wide mortality rate;

12b. age-specific mortality rate for the affected age groups;

12c. sex-specific mortality rates.

Practice Problem Three

During the evening of July 4, a total of 17 people were given emergency treatment at Memorial Hospital for a condition diagnosed as staphylococcal intoxication. Interviews with the people led to identification of an additional 39 people who were ill with signs of staphylococcal intoxication but who did not seek medical attention. Further investigation revealed that all of those ill persons and 42 others (for a total of 98 people) who did not become ill had attended a luncheon at Professor Bonehead's house on July 4. Fourteen of those ill and 37 of those well were females.

13. What is the attack rate of staphylococcal intoxication among the group that attended the picnic?

14. Calculate the sex-specific attack rates.

15. Calculate the ratio of the rate of males to the rate of females.

The age group distribution of the ill and well people is shown in table 5.4.

16. Calculate the age-specific attack rates for each of the age groups shown in the table.

Upon questioning, 53 of the ill people and 3 of the well people could definitely remember that they had eaten the famous Bonehead potato salad that had been prepared several days in advance of the picnic at Professor Bonehead's nonair-

Table 5.4. Cases of Staphylococcal Intoxication, by Age Group

Age Group	No. Ill	No. Well
0–9	0	13
10–19	2	14
20–29	17	10
30–39	24	4
40+	13	1
Total	56	42

conditioned, refrigeratorless kitchen. All other people at the picnic denied having eaten any potato salad.

17. Calculate the food-specific attack rate for those who ate potato salad.

Practice Problem Four

During 1988, a total of 666 cases of dingleitis was reported from a community having a population of 30,000.

18. Calculate the rate of dingleitis in the community during 1988.

Of the 666 cases of dingleitis, 218 occurred during the period of January through March; 61 occurred during the period of April through June; 255 during July through September; and 132 during October through December.

19. Calculate the rates per 10,000 population for dingleitis for each of the quarterly periods.

Further investigation of the 666 cases of dingleitis revealed that 476 cases involved males and the rest females. The number of males in the community was 14,200.

20. Using the rates figured in question 20, determine the ratio of male cases to female cases and the ratio of male rate to the female rate.

21. Calculate the sex-specific disease rates per 10,000 population.

Another item of information obtained during the investigation was the age of the person who had the disease. This information was tabulated by age group and is presented in table 5.5. Also given is the total number of people in each of these age groups who lived in the community.

22. Calculate the age-specific disease rates per 1,000 population for each of the age groups shown above.

Table 5.5. Cases of Dingleitis, by Age Group

Age Group	No. of Cases	Population
0–9	100	7,800
10–19	99	6,500
20–29	65	7,600
30–39	459	4,200
40+	243	3,900
Total	666	30,000

One hundred seventy-five of the 666 cases died. One hundred ten were less than 7 years old and 65 were over 50 years old. One hundred twenty-five were females and 50 were males.

23. Calculate the following mortality rate per 100,000 population:

23a. community-wide mortality rate;

23b. age-specific mortality rate for the affected age groups;

23c. sex-specific mortality rates.

Answers to Practice Problems

1. The rate equals 241/40,000 × base: .006025 × base = 6 per 1,000; 60 per 10,000; 602.50 per 100,000; 6,025 per 1,000,000.

2. For January through March, 44 cases occurred: thus, 44/40,000 × 10,000 (base) = 11 per 10,000. For April through June, 61 cases took place: thus, 61/40,000 × 10,000 = 15.25 per 10,000. For July through September, 0 cases occurred; thus, 0/40,000 × 10,000 = 0 per 10,000. For October through December, 136 cases occurred: thus, 136/40,000 × 10,000 = 34 per 10,000.

3. The key numbers to remember are 76 male cases and 18,500 males in the community. There are also 165 female cases and 21,500 females in the community. To find the male-specific disease rate: 76/18,500 × 10,000 (base) = 41.10 per 10,000 males suffering from computeritis; to find the female specific disease rate: 165/21,500 × 10,000 (base) = 76.70 per 10,000 females in the community suffering from computeritis.

4. To find the ratio of male cases to female cases, you first list the numbers: 76 males; 165 females. The ratio of cases is 76/165 = .46 males to 1.00 female. The ratio of male rate to female rate is 41.10 (males)/76.70 (females) + .54 males to 1.00 female. This means that based on the rate of

10,000 people, for every 1.00 female suffering from computeritis, there are .46 males.

5. You first have to determine the total population of the community (the total population is 40,000). For the 0–9 age group, the rate is 12/6,800 = 1.76 per 1,000. What this means is that for every 1,000 individuals between the ages of 0–9, 1.76 are suffering from computeritis. For the age group 10–19, the formula is 41/8,400 × 1,000 = 4.90 per 1,000; for 20–29, the formula is 62/5,600 × 1,000 = 11.10 per 1,000; for 30–39, the formula is 71/5,200 × 1,000 = 13.70 per 1,000; for 40+, the formula is 55/14,000 × 1,000 = 3.90 per 1,000.

6a. Fifteen individuals died in a population of 40,000, so the formula is 15/40,000 × 100,000 (base) = 37.50 per 100,000 population.

6b. Note that the age group listed in the table is a broad range from 0–9 and that the individuals who were over 50 that died would fall into the 40+ category. So, for the individuals under 9 who died, you had 6 (those that died)/6,800 (population of age group) × 100,000 (base) = 88.20. What this means is that for every 100,000 individuals between 0–9, 88.20 would die from computeritis. For the 10–19, 20–29, and 30–39, all of the mortality rates would be 0 per 100,000, because no one in those age groups died. For the 40+, 9 died, so the formula would be 9/14,000 × 100,000 = 64.30 per 100,000.

6c. Eight females died, and the community consisted of 21,500 females. Seven males died, and the community consisted of 18,500 males. To get the female-specific mortality rate: 8/21,500 × 100,000 = 37.20 per 100,000 females dying from computeritis. To get the male-specific mortality rate: 7/18,500 × 100,000 = 37.80 per 100,000 males dying from computeritis.

7. Rate of SLD: 126/20,000 × base = 6.30 per 1,000, or 63 per 10,000, or 630 per 100,000.

8. For the period of January through March, 0 per 10,000; for April through June, 5/20,000 × 10,000 = 2.50 per 10,000; for July through September, 113/20,000 × 10,000 = 56.50 per 10,000; for October through December, 8/20,000 × 10,000 = 4 per 10,000.

9. Of the 126 cases, 67 were males and 59 cases were female. There were 9,200 males and 10,800 females. The male rate is 67/9,200 × 10,000 = 72.80 per 10,000; the female rate is 59/10,800 × 10,000 = 54.60 per 10,000.

10. The ratio of male cases to female cases is 67/59 = 1.14 males to 1.00 female; the ratio of male rate to female rate is 72.80/54.60 = 1.33 males to 1.00 female.

11. For the 0–9 age group, 17/3,400 × 1,000 = 5 per 1,000; for 10–19, 18/4,200 × 1,000 = 4.30 per 1,000; for 20–29, 9/2,800 × 1,000 = 3.20 per

1,000; for 30–39, 11/2,600 × 1,000 = 4.20 per 1,000; for 40+, 71/7,000 × 1,000 = 10.10 per 1,000.

12a. The rate is 4/20,000 × 100,000 = 20 per 100,000.

12b. For the 0–9 age group, 1/3,400 × 100,000 = 29.40 per 100,000; for 10–19, 20–29, and 30–39, the age-specific mortality rate is 0; for 40+, 3/7,000 × 100,000 = 42.90 per 100,000.

12c. Two males died, out of a population of 9,200 males: thus, 2/9,200 × 100,000 = 21.70 per 100,000 males; 2 females died, out of 10,800 females: thus, 2/10,800 × 100,000 = 18.50 per 100,000 females.

13. Let's reiterate the numbers: 56 people were ill and 42 were well; of the ill people, 14 were females and 42 were males; of the 42 well people, 5 were males and 37 were females. Of the 98 people, 51 were females and 47 were males. Of the 98 people that attended the picnic, 56 were ill, so 56/98 × base (100) = 57.10 per 100 people is the attack rate.

14. Sex-specific attack rate: 42 males/47 total males × 100 = 89.40 per 100 males; 14 females/51 total females × 100 = 27.50 per 100 females.

15. The rate of males is 89.40 and the rate of females is 27.50; the ratio of male rate to female rate is 89.40/27.50 = 3.25 to 1.00 (for ever 1.00 female, 3.25 males become ill).

16. For the 0–9 age group, the rate is 0; for 10–19, the rate is 2/16 × base (100) = 12.50 per 100; for 20–29, 17/27 × base = 63 per 100; for 30–39, 24/28 × base = 85.70 per 100; for 40+, 13/14 × base = 92.90 per 100.

17. Of the 56 that ate the potato salad, 53 became ill, so the rate would be 53/56 × base (100) = 94.60 per 100. So, for every 100 people who ate potato salad, 94.60 became ill.

18. The rate is 666/30,000 × base (1,000) = 22.20 per 1,000.

19. For January through March, 218/30,000 × 10,000 = 72.70; for April through June, 61/30,000 × 10,000 – 20.30; for July through September, 255/30,000 × 10,000 = 85; for October through December, 132/30,000 × 10,000 = 44.

20. Of the 666 cases, 476 were males and 190 were females. The male population is 14,200 and the female population is 15,800, so the male rate is 476/14,200 × 10,000 = 335.20; the female rate is 190/15,800 × 10,000 = 120.30.

21. The ratio of male cases to female cases is 476/190 = 2.50 males to 1.00 female. The ratio of male rate to female rate is 335.20/120.3 = 2.79 males to 1.00 female.

22. For the 0–9 age group, 100/7,800 × 1,000 = 12.80; for 10–19, 99/6,500 ×

1,000 = 15.20; for 20–29, 65/7,600 × 1,000 = 8.60; for 30–39, 159/4,200 × 1,000 = 37.90; for 40+, 243/3,900 × 1,000 = 62.30.

23a. The rate is 175/30,000 × 100,000 = 583.30.

23b. For the 0–9 age group, 110/7,800 × 100,000 = 1,410.25; for 10–19, 20–29, and 30–39 the rate is 0; for 40+, 65/3,900 × 100,000 = 1,674.40.

23c. For males, 50/14,200 × 100,000 = 352.10; for females, 125/15,800 × 100,000 = 791.10.

6

Standardization of
Vital Statistics

In chapter 5 I touched briefly on the possibility of comparing two different populations by "adjusting" or "standardizing" the rates. This chapter will provide information needed to understand standardization and then will discuss the techniques used to compare populations.

First, you probably don't need to adjust rates if two communities are similar. Whether or not the communities are similar is a judgment of the vital statistician performing the study. Determinants could include the ratio of various ethnic groups and the *enumerated* (actual count) populations of various age groups. For example, if you are looking at two counties, both with a population of fifty thousand equally distributed among age groups and a similar proportion of ethnic groups, then you don't need to adjust rates. You can compare the communities with the various crude and specific rate processes.

However, in many instances the vital statistician may be comparing very different communities. Adjusting rates allows a person to compare on equal terms. First, I need to point out that adjusted or standardized rates are *artificial rates*. They are not intended to represent a community but are merely used for comparison purposes.

One of the first things a vital statistician needs to do prior to figuring any standardization rate is to find a *standard population*. A standard population is a population to which both communities are compared. Keep in mind that there are no right or wrong standard populations; it is a technique to help the vital statistician compare two communities. A good standard population to use is the United States standard population found in the U.S. Census data. A little investigation among the government documents section of a library will reveal this information. The actual population figures of groups are referred to as *enumerated populations*. Appendix B of this book lists the 1990 U.S. Census enumerated populations of various age groups. With this type information, one can compare whatever age groups one studies in the vital statistics.

A second commonly used standard population type is the *pooled population*, which is the combined population of both communities. This technique is useful when you do not have access to any other standard population.

Table 6.1. Enumerated Populations in Selected Age Groups, 1990 Census

Age Group	Enumerated Population
0–4	18,354,443
5–14	35,213,128
15–24	36,741,327
25–34	43,175,932
35–44	37,578,908
45–64	46,371,016
65+	31,238,831
Total	248,673,585

A third technique used to present a standard population is to express the *percentage of population*. This is especially useful in multiplying the figures.

Finally, the fourth type of standard population is the *standard million*. This reduces the population to only one million people but keeps all proportions similar to the enumerated populations.

Standard Population Types

There are four major standard population types: enumerated population, standard million, pooled population, and percentage of population. Each of these four requires a special formula.

Enumerated Population

Let's start building our case study for this chapter by first describing the standard population that we will be using. Note, you do not have to use the United States standard population; you can use whichever one you want. However, the United States standard population is the most commonly used.

By looking at the list of numbers in table 6.1, you can see that there are large population numbers listed. According to this list the 1990 United States population had slightly over 248 million people. Dealing with the enumerated populations can be cumbersome, and in many instances your calculator will not be able to handle such large numbers. In order to deal with this more efficiently, one can use the standard million method of expressing standard population.

Standard Million

This technique is one that proportionately reduces the enumerated population of each age group so that the total population equals one million. This process is relatively simple. First, you need the total population in each respective age category. You also need to know the total standard population you are using. Let's say that the United States population of those under age five consisted of 18,354,443 people, out of a total of 248,673,580. Divide 18,354,443 by 248,673,580 and then multiply by 1,000,000. Let's take that step by step:

$$18,354,443 \div 248,673,580 = .07380938$$
$$.07380938 \times 1,000,000 = 73,809$$

You proceed to do this with each age group. So, what does this mean? Well, imagine a mysterious virus from outer space infected the United States, and it proportionately reduced the United States population to just one million people. Of these one million people, 73,809 would be in the age category 0–4. Complete the rest of the following table based on the 1990 census. The answers can be found in table B.2 in Appendix B.

Age Group	Enumerated Population	Standard Million
0–4	18,354,443	73,809
5–9	18,099,179	
10–14	17,113,949	
15–19	17,721,015	
20–24	19,020,312	
25–29	21,313,045	
30–34	21,862,887	
35–44	37,578,903	
45–54	25,223,086	
55–64	21,147,930	
65+	31,238,831	
Total	248,673,580	

After you finish this task, keep this information available. The United States standard million is probably the most commonly used standard population type in vital statistics. By the way, more specific information on the United States 1990 populations can be found in tables B.1 and B.2 in Appendix B.

Pooled Population

The pooled population is a combination of two populations, to which each specific community is then compared. The idea behind this approach is that any biases are neutralized by the stability of both communities. Also, it's relatively simple to do, especially if you do not access to a United States standard population or standard million. An example of this type will be given later in the chapter.

Percentage of Standard Population

To figure the percentage of the standard population of various age groups, divide the enumerated population of the age group by the total population and multiply by

Table 6.2. Age-Specific Death Rates of Robbyville and Carlyville

Age Group	Robbyville			Carlyville		
	No. of Deaths	Population	ASDR°	No. of Deaths	Population	ASDR°
0–4	150	35,000	428.57	25	5,000	500.00
5–14	95	140,000	67.86	9	15,000	60.00
15–24	125	160,000	78.13	5	35,000	14.29
25–34	70	140,000	50.00	15	30,000	50.00
35–44	45	100,000	45.00	35	25,000	140.00
45–64	150	75,000	200.00	100	20,000	500.00
65+	300	55,000	545.45	125	15,000	833.33
Total	935	705,000	132.62	314	145,000	216.55

°Rate per 100,000

100. It makes for very easy calculations. Table B.2 shows the percentage of population of the various age groups.

Direct Method of Adjusting

The direct method of adjusting is a technique in which you use the actual age-specific death rates of two or more communities. This is the only method of adjusting that we will discuss. The indirect method of adjusting is needed when you do not have access to those age-specific death rates; it is more complicated and not commonly used by vital statisticians outside the federal government.

After you have selected the standard population, you can now make comparisons. Generally speaking, most people do not use the enumerated population as their standard population because of the large numbers that are involved. Thus, for the sake of this book, we will only focus on the standard million, percentage, or pooled population as our standard populations. After you select one of these standard population types, you then need to compute the age-specific rate for each community you are studying. In this particular example, we are going to examine the death rates of Robbyville and Carlyville. Table 6.2 shows the age-specific death rates.

Using the Standard Million Population

After you complete the age-specific death rates (ASDR), you can incorporate this data into a table with the United States standard million population.

The ASDRs of Robbyville and Carlyville are reported in table 6.3. The expected deaths are what one would expect if the age populations were distributed like that of the United States. The purpose of adjusting these rates is to control for the unique differences between the two communities. For example, in table 6.2, it appears that the age distribution of Robbyville is slanted toward the older populations, whereas Carlyville's age distribution leans toward the younger age groups. Thus, one would expected a

Table 6.3. Expected Deaths in Robbyville and Carlyville, by Age Group (Using 1990 U.S. Standard Million Population)

Column	1	2	3	4	5
		Robbyville		Carlyville	
Age Group	1990 U.S. Standard Million	ASDR	Expected Deaths	ASDR	Expected Deaths
0–4	73,809	428.57		500.00	
5–14	141,604	67.86		60.00	
15–24	102,736	78.13		14.29	
25–34	173,625	50.00		50.00	
35–44	151,117	45.00		140.00	
45–64	186,473	200.00		500.00	
65+	170,636	545.45		833.33	
Total	1,000,000	132.62		216.55	

higher death rate for Robbyville. Yet, if one looks at the data in table 6.2 it appears that Carlyville has a higher death rate. By adjusting the data into *expected deaths*, we remove the effects of certain variables that can adversely affect the rates. It's important to remember that these expected deaths are artificial rates.

In order to get the expected deaths for Robbyville, you first multiply the standard million population in column 1 times the Robbyville ASDR (column 2) and then divide that result by 1,000,000. To get the expected deaths for Carlyville, you multiply the population in column 1 times the Carlyville ASDR (column 4) and divide by 1,000,000. Complete the expected deaths for Robbyville and Carlyville and then check the results in table 6.3A.

From the results, you can now make comparisons that are free from those unique variables that can bias a certain community. A closer examination of Robbyville and Carlyville reveals that very little difference exists between the expected deaths of 0–14 and the 25–34 age groups. Carlyville has a larger increase of expected deaths for those individuals 35 and older. On the other hand, the expected deaths were almost six times higher in Robbyville than in Carlyville in the 15–24 age group. Also, Carlyville's expected deaths were three times that of Robbyville's in the 35–44 and 45–64 age groups and not quite double that of the 65 and over group. Note that the formula would be identical if you were to use the enumerated population instead of the standard million. But your calculations would be so difficult to determine that you would probably resort to an abbreviated standard population such as the standard million.

Using Pooled Population

Let's take the same information from table 6.2; but instead of using the standard million population we are going to combine the populations of Robbyville and Carlyville. Table 6.4 represents the new data.

Remember, you received individual populations of Robbyville and Carlyville in

Table 6.3A. Expected Deaths in Robbyville and Carlyville, by Age Group (Using 1990 U.S. Standard Million Population)—Answers

Column	1	2	3	4	5
		Robbyville		Carlyville	
Age Group	1990 U.S. Standard Million	ASDR	Expected Deaths	ASDR	Expected Deaths
0–4	73,809	428.57	31.63	500.00	36.90
5–14	141,604	67.86	9.61	60.00	8.50
15–24	102,736	78.13	8.03	14.29	1.47
25–34	173,625	50.00	8.68	50.00	8.68
35–44	151,117	45.00	6.80	140.00	21.16
45–64	186,473	200.00	37.29	500.00	93.24
65+	170,636	545.45	93.07	833.33	142.20
Total	1,000,000	132.62	195.12	216.55	312.14

table 6.2, and in this table you combine the two populations. This is called a pooled population. Your age-specific death rates (ASDR) are also taken from table 6.2. To get the expected deaths, you follow the procedure similar to that used with the standard million population. You multiply the ASDR (columns 2 and 4) times the pooled population for that age group (column 1) and then you divide by the total population—in this case, 850,000.

Using Percentage of Standard Population

Once again, let's take the information from table 6.2 and use the percentage of the enumerated population to figure the expected deaths, as demonstrated in table 6.5.

With this approach you multiply the age group percentage of population (column 1) times the ASDR (columns 2 and 4) to find the expected deaths. For example, for Robbyville's 0–4 age group, you would multiply 428.57 times 7.38% (or .0738) to get 31.63 expected deaths. Remember, the numbers in the expected deaths columns (3 and 5), regardless of the type of standard population, are artificial data and intended for comparison purposes only. Note that the expected death results look very familiar to those given in table 6.4 using the standard million population. That is because you have used proportionately similar numbers (standard million and percentage). The differences are only due to the fact that in a standard million you are dealing with five or six digits, whereas in the standard percentage, you are dealing with primarily two digits (and up to two decimal places).

Finally, we need to talk about why one would standardize. Part of the reason for standardization is to ensure political correctness. Let me try to explain this. For those of you who are aware of research methods, you know that the sampling of your population is extremely important. If you do a *random selection*, what you are basically saying is that you are willing to bet that the sample you draw from this random process will represent your total population. Basically, statistical odds do show that you are very likely to have

Table 6.4. Expected Deaths in Robbyville and Carlyville, by Age Group (Using Pooled Population)

Column	1	2	3	4	5
		Robbyville		Carlyville	
Age Group	Pooled Population	ASDR	Expected Deaths	ASDR	Expected Deaths
0–4	40,000	428.57	20.17	500.00	23.53
5–14	155,000	67.86	12.37	60.00	10.94
15–24	195,000	78.13	17.92	14.29	3.28
25–34	170,000	50.00	10.00	50.00	10.00
35–44	125,000	45.00	6.62	140.00	20.59
45–64	95,000	200.00	22.35	500.00	55.88
65+	70,000	545.45	44.92	833.33	68.63
Total	850,000				

a sample that represents your overall population. For example, if you have 55% Catholics in your population, a random selection will represent very close to 55% Catholics. It may not be exactly 55%, and if you were to do this random selection many times, you would note that this number can vary dramatically. Yet, from a research method standpoint, random selection is appropriate.

Occasionally, researchers may want to do a *stratified random selection*. The idea behind this is to ensure that various subgroups are appropriately represented. If you had a community of ten thousand residents, with nine thousand whites and one thousand blacks, your random selection process should give you approximately the same proportion of whites and blacks. Yet it's possible you might come up with a higher proportion of whites in your sample than in the community. In order to avoid this, researchers will do a stratified random selection process. This is where the researcher breaks the population into various subgroups (e.g., whites and blacks) and then proceeds to randomly select the appropriate number from each group. For example, if you have ten thousand residents, of which 90% are white and the rest are black, and if you want a sample of one thousand, the researcher would separate whites from blacks and choose 10% of each group. Thus, you would get nine hundred whites and one hundred blacks.

Now, why would somebody do something like this? If you are planning a program for a community that has a wide range of cultural and ethnic differences, you would want your "sample" to represent your community. Now, theoretically, if you did a random selection, you would have equal proportions. But it's possible that this random process would give you a higher proportion of one group than another. For example, let's go back to our earlier example of ten thousand residents, with nine thousand whites and one thousand blacks. Suppose you did a "random" selection of one thousand, and let's say you get nine thousand, five hundred whites and five hundred blacks. Theoretically, this is a sufficient sample, yet if you try to convince a group of community black leaders about the results, they may question if your sample properly represents the black com-

Table 6.5. Expected Deaths in Robbyville and Carlyville, by Age Group
(Using Percentage of Population)

Column	1	2	3	4	5
		Robbyville		Carlyville	
Age Group	Percentage of U.S. Population	ASDR[°]	Expected Deaths	ASDR[°]	Expected Deaths
0–4	7.38	428.57	31.63	500.00	36.90
5–14	14.28	67.86	9.69	60.00	8.57
15–24	14.78	78.13	11.55	14.29	2.11
25–34	17.36	50.00	8.68	50.00	8.68
35–44	15.11	45.00	6.80	140.00	21.15
45–64	18.64	200.00	37.28	500.00	93.20
65+	12.56	545.45	68.51	833.33	104.67
Total	100.11[a]				

[a] Total may not equal 100% due to rounding up of figures

[°] Rate per 100,000

munity. So a stratified random selection ensures that you will have the same proportion of blacks in your sample as there are in the community.

Now, what does this have to do with standardizing vital statistics. As with stratified random selection, standardizing data may also help you politically. If you try to compare Chicago to Carbondale, Illinois, even if you use rates, people may argue that you cannot compare a large metropolitan city to a rural community. By standardizing, you attempt to balance and equalize differences in populations. Thus the standardized rate differences of the communities you are comparing may not be that much different from the raw rates, but standardization represents an attempt to offset major differences between the communities.

7

Decision Making in
Public Health

How do you make a decision? Oftentimes the decision many of us make seems almost like an instinct. We automatically reach for our toothbrushes when we get up in the morning or when we're ready to go to bed. We automatically turn the coffee on when we walk into the kitchen in the morning. Some may argue that these are not decisions but rather automated activities. Regardless, an important part of a decision is an action. This chapter will discuss two very important tools that help vital statisticians make decisions: the two by two table and the decision tree.

Two by Two Table

Before we talk about the decision-making model, I would like to describe a very popular and important table—the two by two table. As you become more adept at using vital statistics and understanding the basic concepts of epidemiology (the study of disease), this table will become more and more important.

There are four squares in the two by two table, indicating there are four possible options: true positive, false positive, true negative, and false negative. The two by two table gives a person a pictorial view of the four options: two that provide accurate information and two that provide false information. It is important to know the potential errors associated with certain processes or tests. For example, home pregnancy tests are very popular and affordable. Yet how accurate are they? According to the test, a woman is either pregnant or not pregnant. On a two by two table, the presence of a condition or a disease (e.g., pregnancy, cancer) is reflected in the columns. On the top of the two by two table the event is identified as being present or absent. Using our example of a pregnancy, you will note in table 7.1 that the left column states pregnancy is present while the right column states pregnancy is absent.

The left side of the two by two table describes the results of the pregnancy test. Either the test will reveal that a woman is pregnant or it will reveal that she is not pregnant. The four squares are representative of the four options. If a woman is pregnant and the test shows that she is pregnant, then it's considered a *true positive* test. If she is pregnant but the test shows that she is not pregnant, then it's considered a *false nega-*

Table 7.1. Status of Pregnancy Two by Two Table

Test Results	Status of Pregnancy	
	Pregnancy Is Present	Pregnancy Is Absent
Pregnancy Test Is Positive	true positive	false positive
Pregnancy Test Is Negative	false negative	true negative

tive. False in that the result is incorrect and *negative* in the sense that negative (in medical terms) indicates nothing is wrong.

If she is not pregnant and the pregnancy test comes back positive, then it is considered a *false positive* test. *False*, as indicated before, in that it is incorrect, whereas *positive* is indicative of something taking place. Finally, if she is not pregnant and the test reveals a negative result (indicating that she is not pregnant), then the result is referred to as a *true negative*.

Of the four squares, one would hope that the true positive and the true negative would be the only two results. Unfortunately, that does not always take place. A number of factors can account for a person receiving a false negative or a false positive. A false negative might occur if a woman takes the home pregnancy examination too early in her pregnancy and the woman's body is not producing sufficient levels of the human chorionic gonadotropin (HCG) hormone. A false positive test might result if the urine is collected in a contaminated container or if she has taken some medication or another drug the day before. Regardless of the reason, both the false negative and the false positive can lead to some dangerous consequences. For example, if the woman is pregnant and her examination shows that she is not (false negative), she might inadvertently take some drug that could cause damage to the embryo. On the other hand, imagine the potential despair of a woman who is told that she is pregnant when in reality she isn't (false positive).

There are many health-related issues that can incorporate the two by two table. Any clinical test has the potential of error, for example, the test for HIV. As health-care costs become more and more expensive, it will become increasingly more important for health-care workers to utilize those tests that have the greatest potential for a correct diagnosis. The idea of the two by two table is to identify the potential risks or errors in many types of tests.

In public health and in many clinical settings, certain terms are used to discuss the potential errors that might exist with various tests. As the discussion of the two by two table advances, you will note that there will be numbers listed in each of the four squares. These numbers may be represented in raw figures, percentages, or proportions. The terms relating to the two by two table include sensitivity, specificity, positive predictive value, and negative predictive value. First, let's talk about sensitivity and specificity.

Sensitivity

Sensitivity is the measurement of the ability of any clinical test to detect a disease

Table 7.2. Status of Diabetes Two by Two Table

Test Results	Status of Diabetes	
	Diabetes Is Present (Sensitivity)	Diabetes Is Absent (Specificity)
Test Is Positive	true positive	false positive
Test Is Negative	false negative	true negative

when the disease is present. Obviously, if you had diabetes, you would hope that the test the physician performs on you would detect that disease. The closer to 100%, the better. Keep in mind that there are few, if any, tests that are 100% effective. On a two by two table, sensitivity is reflected in the column on the left side, under the section entitled disease positive or present. This column lists the actual number of cases of a disease.

Specificity

Specificity is the measurement of the ability of a test to determine that a person doesn't have a disease when the disease is absent. Imagine the dismay you would experience if a test indicated that you were a diabetic when in reality you were not a diabetic. Specificity is the ability of the test to identify those individuals who don't have the disease and is located on the right-side column of the two by two table under the section listed disease negative or not present.

Let's set up an imaginary study on a two by two table. Imagine that you tested for diabetes one thousand people who were representative of the total population. Table 7.2 is an example of a basic two by two table showing a diabetes study. On the very top you will see the heading Actual Presence of Diabetes, and above the left column you note the statement Diabetes Is Present. On the right column you will note the statement Diabetes Is Absent. The left column is reflective of all the diabetics, whereas the right column is reflective of all nondiabetics.

On the left side of the two by two table, you will note the heading Test Results, with a positive designation on the top row and a negative designation on the bottom row. Those are the two possible reactions that you will get from your test—either positive or negative.

Imagine now that you have a special test called a Diabetes Test Finder to determine whether a person is a diabetic. Your Diabetes Test Finder will not be perfect but then there are very few tests that are 100% accurate or that have sensitivity or specificity of 100%. Table 7.3 shows the results of your diabetes testing.

Now, remember that you are testing one thousand individuals representative of the total population. From previous investigations, you already know that 5% of the population is diabetic. So of these one thousand people, you know that you have fifty diabetics. Note where the number 50 is placed on table 7.3. It is placed at the bottom of the left column indicating all actual cases.

If you have fifty diabetics from a sample of one thousand, then you will have nine hundred fifty people who are not diabetics. Note that the 950 is placed at the bottom of

Table 7.3. Results of the Diabetes Test Finder

Test Results	Actual Presence of Diabetes		Total
	Diabetes Is Present (sensitivity = .80)	Diabetes Is Absent (specificity = .90)	
Test Is Positive	40 (true positive)	95 (false positive)	135
Test Is Negative	10 (false negative)	855 (true negative)	865
Total Cases	50	950	1,000

the right column. Remember the right column are those individuals who do not have the disease.

But what about the numbers in the actual squares? For example, if you were to test these one thousand people with the Diabetes Test Finder, how many would be in the four categories of true positive, false positive, false negative, and true negative? This is where the sensitivity and specificity of the test is used. Sensitivity and specificity are numbers that are provided to medical workers by the company that provides the laboratory test.

If the sensitivity of the Diabetes Test Finder is .80, you would multiply the sensitivity by the total number of diabetics in the population (50), which was determined by the prevalence of the disease (remember, we said that this sample is representative of the total population and that 5% of the population is diabetic). If you multiply the sensitivity and the total number of diabetics (.80 sensitivity times 50 diabetics), you see that forty individuals tested who had the disease would test positive. Thus, the 40 is placed in the upper left corner, while 10 would be placed in the lower left corner (50 minus 40). The lower left corner is the false negative section, meaning that ten individuals who are diabetics would receive a test indicating that they do not have the disease.

Now, how about the column on the right side? This lists the individuals who do not have diabetes. Again, some of these individuals will receive accurate results (true negative), whereas some others will receive false information (false positive).

Since you know from earlier discussions that 950 individuals are not diabetics, you can multiply that number and the specificity to determine the true negative results (lower-right corner). Let's say the specificity of the Diabetes Test Finder is .90. Multiply .90 times 950, and you'll find that 855 of the 950 nondiabetics would receive a true negative test (thus, 855 is placed in the lower-right corner). Subtract 855 from 950, and you'll find that 95 individuals would receive false positives (upper right-hand corner). These are the individuals who do not have diabetes but who would test positive; thus, they receive a false positive.

If you total the rows, you will come up with 1,000 (the total of the sample), because everyone is accounted for in the rows. Also, if you add the two columns, they will total 1,000. These are the self-checks to make sure that you did your math correctly. The beauty of the two by two table is that if you have some of the numbers, you can figure out the others.

Predictive Value

There are two more terms that you need to be familiar with. These are the *positive predictive values* and the *negative predictive values*. Sensitivity and specificity are useful measures of how efficient a test is, but their calculation requires that you know the patient's true condition. If you know for sure whether the patient is diseased or not, why do the test? Thus, in clinical studies, a person is more interested in the *predictive value* of the test. Predictive value is another tool that vital statisticians can use to make decisions. It is a proportion that can help the epidemiologist and clinical worker make appropriate decisions.

Positive Predictive Value

The positive predictive value (PPV) is determined by adding the true positives and false positives and dividing the true positives by the total positives. With our diabetes example, the true positives are 40 and the false positives are 95. Add the two together to total 135. Divide the true positives (40) by the total number of positive tests (135) to get a positive predictive value of .2963. That means that of all the positive results of the Diabetes Test Finder, only 29.63% of the positive tests will be of true diabetics.

Negative Predictive Value

The negative predictive value (NPV) is determined in similar fashion. Add the false negatives and the true negatives. In this case, you have 10 false negatives plus 855 true negatives, which total 865. Divide the true negatives by the total number of negative results. Thus, you divide 855 by 865 to get .9884. This means that of all of the negative results, 98.84% will be of true nondiabetics.

Based on these numbers, what does this say about the Diabetes Test Finder? Well, it says that if one doesn't have diabetes, it is a very accurate test. On the other hand, if one does have diabetes, there's less than a one out of three chance that the test will indicate that. In other words, a positive test on the Diabetes Test Finder is far from conclusive, and further tests need to be conducted. However, if the test reveals a negative result, there's a very good chance (98.84%) that the person doesn't have diabetes. It's a good screening device to determine if a person is a nondiabetic but a relatively poor determining test of a diabetic.

Keep in mind that all we are talking about is probability. It's entirely possible that these numbers may be altered slightly, because in real life we do have variations. These tables are merely tools to help public health officials, epidemiologists, and clinical personnel make decisions and/or identify problems.

A Real-Life Situation

Imagine that you are working in a public health department in a midwestern state of four and one-half million people. The state has been characterized as white collar and agricultural with most people working in service, research, and development industries. The unemployment rate is 4.5%. Ten percent of the population is retired, and one-third is below eighteen years of age.

The state legislature is quite concerned about the AIDS epidemic and wants to

Table 7.4. First ELISA Test for HIV

| | Actual Presence of HIV | | |
| | HIV Is Present | HIV Is Absent | |
Test Results	(sensitivity = .998)	(specificity = .983)	Total
Test Is Positive	699 (true positive)	16,988 (false positive)	17,687
Test Is Negative	1 (false negative)	982,312 (true negative)	982,313
Total Cases	700	999,300	1,000,000

institute mandatory HIV testing of all state employees, applicants for marriage licenses, food handlers, health-care workers, all people arrested, teachers, college students, patients admitted to hospitals, prisoners, and people receiving public assistance. Approximately one million people would be directly affected by this program. The governor disagrees with this plan. Both parties wish to avoid a public confrontation on this issue, so they call upon the apolitical public health department to provide guidance. You are given the responsibility of developing the policy.

You decide to plot two by two tables to determine of the one million people who would be eligible for the HIV testing how many would receive true positive, false positive, true negative, and false negative results. As you are aware, HIV is detected by two clinical blood tests. The first test, the ELISA, will show a positive result if there is the presence of the antibodies that HIV produces (as you may be aware, we cannot test for the actual virus that causes AIDS, only its antibody). The ELISA antibody test is conducted twice. If both tests come back positive, then a Western Blot (WB) antibody test is given. The Western Blot is very accurate (and it is also very expensive, thus it is used only after two ELISA positive test results). The sensitivity of ELISA is .998 and the specificity is .983. The sensitivity of the Western Blot is 1.00 and the specificity is .944. In this particular state, the incidence of HIV is .70 per 1,000. Thus, one can expect to have 700 individuals with HIV among these 1,000,000 tests, as demonstrated in table 7.4.

Your first ELISA test would reveal what? (Note, all numbers are rounded up.) Your first ELISA test reveals that 17,687 may be infected with HIV. Of course, your superior training reminds you that there are some false positives associated with the test, so you redo the ELISA test with those 17,687 positive tests—because you do not know at this time which of the 17,687 are true positives and which are false positives (see table 7.5).

Now you have 987 individuals who have tested positive for HIV. There are still some false readings, but you hope that the Western Blot will reduce those even more. Incorporating the sensitivity (1.00) and specificity (.944) of the Western Blot, table 7.6 shows the results of the WB test on those 987 individuals.

Now 16 of the 714 positive Western Blot tests are false positives. Divide 700 true positives by 716 and you will get a positive predictive value of 97.8% for your initial one million cases. This example should show you how you proceed from one step to another.

Thus, for the one million individuals you are testing for HIV, you will ultimately discover 700 individuals who will be given a true positive result and 16 who will falsely

Table 7.5. Second ELISA Test for HIV

Test Results	Actual Presence of HIV		Total
	HIV Is Present (sensitivity = .998)	HIV Is Absent (specificity = .983)	
Test Is Positive	699 (true positive)	288 (false positive)	987
Test Is Negative	1 (false negative)	16,699 (true negative)	16,700
Total Cases	700	16,987	17,687

be identified as having HIV. As you prepare your report to the governor, you will need to consider other issues such as costs of these exams and whether such costs would outweigh your decision to test everyone. At this time, most public health officials feel that the cost, inconvenience of testing, and the small number of HIV-infected individuals far outweigh the need to mass test populations such as illustrated in this example.

Decision Tree

Think of decisions you make in your professional life. In many instances (perhaps more times than you realize), your decisions are based on probabilities. A decision you make is based on the odds of something happening. For example, if you have a choice between two people to hire, you tend to look at their strengths and weaknesses and then you can somewhat assess a "point total." This is basically making a decision based on odds.

Recently, business decisions have been based on the decision-tree model. Even more recently, the medical profession has turned to this model to assist in decisions. Public health officials can also benefit from this model.

This model utilizes a tree format. The "branches" show the results of possible choices of the decision maker. In the tree, there are two types of junctions. A square depicts a decision that needs to be made by the decision maker, and a circle indicates a

Table 7.6. Western Blot Test for HIV

Test Results	Actual Presence of HIV		Total
	HIV Is Present (sensitivity = 1.000)	HIV Is Absent (specificity = .944)	
Test Is Positive	700 (true positive)	16 (false positive)	716
Test Is Negative	0 (false negative)	271 (true negative)	271
Total Cases	700	287	987

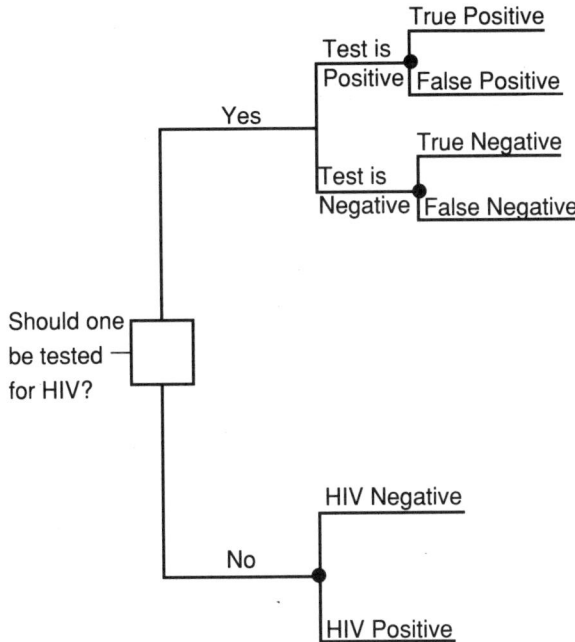

Fig. 7.1. Decision tree on determining appropriateness of testing for HIV

"chance" mode, both of which have more than one option. Our example will just have two options; however, in many instances those options will be greater than two.

Let's walk through a decision-making process. Besides a narrative description, the process will also be plotted on figure 7.1.

Let's use the scenario previously described. The governor has appointed you as the director of your state's public health program. The governor has been under tremendous pressure from certain forces throughout the state to mandate HIV testing for all public workers, which would include teachers, police officers, fire fighters, medical workers, employees in the public health sectors, and basically all individuals who work in any public-related settings. The total of such workers conveniently happens to be one million employees.

The governor doesn't know what to do (sounds familiar, huh?) and has asked you for your ruling. He has indicated that he will abide by your decision. Not wanting to be political, you vow to make a decision based on the "facts." For your decision tree you first need to determine that you have one of two choices (a decision node): you can either test everyone for the HIV antibody or you could not test everyone. As can be seen in figure 7.1, the decision branch to test is on top, whereas the decision branch not to test is on the bottom.

Let's first focus on the bottom branch. Not testing will result in one of two choices—either the individual will be an unknown HIV positive or an unknown HIV negative. In fact, based on the numbers given in the previous scenario, the rate of HIV infection in this particular state is .70/1,000. Thus, if you choose not to test, seven hundred individuals (of this population of one million) will be unaware of their HIV status (of course you realize that some of these individuals will eventually discover the infection on their own).

The top part of the tree is much more complicated. After deciding to test everyone, you will have one of two results—either the tests will reveal that the person is positive or that the person is negative. Note the section in figure 7.1. Just because a person tests positive, it doesn't mean that it's true. For anyone who tests positive, you have one of two results. Either it's a true positive (the person actually does have the antibodies to HIV) or it's a false positive (the test indicates the person is infected when in reality the person does not have the virus)—so that particular junction is a "chance" mode.

For those who were tested and the false reading came up, there are also two possible results. The reading could be accurate, and the negative test accurately reflects that the person does not have the virus. On the other hand, the negative test could be wrong (a false negative), and the person is actually infected but the test doesn't show it yet (a legitimate concern since HIV has a seroconversion of six weeks to six months after initial infection).

So there you have it: the complete tree of the decision to test all public employees for HIV. But how does this help a person make a decision? Well, first of all it's helpful just to look at the various options. In addition, you can insert the figures you've worked out on the practice two by two tables you completed earlier in this chapter. At the upper right section of the tree, start putting in the appropriate numbers for the true positives, true negatives, false positives, and the false negatives.

By doing some "folding" and "pruning," one is able to determine the probability of whether to test these one million people. Based on the numbers, the probability would be best not to test everyone for HIV.

There are many books that have been written on this topic, and it is difficult to condense the major ideas into just one chapter. The decision tree is a device to help the clinician make decisions. It shouldn't be the sole factor, but it's an attempt to prevent bias and/or prejudices from getting in the way.

8
Summary

This textbook was written to provide the practicing public health official or other consumer with a better understanding of methods used to interpret vital statistics. As you have seen, figuring statistics is not extremely difficult but it can be confusing. For that reason, it might be best to maintain this book for future reference. Besides providing you with a useful reference tool, it will also allow more people to buy this book new, and from a statistical standpoint, that is significant to me.

The purpose of this chapter is to summarize and to discuss the role in which vital statistics are used in our society. As mentioned in an earlier chapter, it is not unusual for various government organizations to select preliminary sites for programs based solely on information obtained from vital statistics. Those statistics can be based on mortality, morbidity, racial composition, or income disparities. It may not seem fair, but that's the way the game is played.

To summarize:

1. All data that are used by the federal, state, and local governments are available to the public. Almost all are available free of charge and can be obtained by getting on the appropriate mailing list.
2. Remember that data can be manipulated to say anything.
3. If you take the time to collect, interpret, and utilize vital statistics in your daily work environment, you will really impress your boss, co-workers, family, friends, loved ones, and parents. As you can see in reading this book, understanding and utilizing such data does not take a great deal of intelligence, but it does take a great deal of perseverance (also true for writing such a book). Yet it's amazing how many intelligent, well-read individuals look at such data and panic.
4. People can argue philosophies, what should or should not be done and who should do such things, but it is very hard to argue "data." In spite of the fact that unethical people can manipulate data to fit their needs, it nonetheless is very difficult to argue with "facts." Thus, the ability to interpret vital statistics is a very important tool in combating groups who have philosophically different viewpoints. For example, there are many different views on what should be done regarding adolescent pregnancies. Yet no one can argue statistics that report on the rate, proportion, or ratio of these pregnancies. While everyone is arguing philosophy, you can calmly report data. Eventually, because you have the facts, people will turn to you for your opinion on what should be done.

5. Be critical of reports you read that use tables, graphs, and other data. Keep in mind that the person writing the information may not understand the data he/she is discussing. Be a wise consumer of vital statistics.

I hope that this textbook can be of some value to you. It's relatively small and simplistic, yet it contains important concepts concerning vital statistics that all too often are not discussed at length. In preparing for the writing of this text, I found that most information about vital statistics is included in regular statistics textbooks or imbedded in the introductory chapters of epidemiology books. What makes vital statistics so frightening for so many people is their lack of confidence in the use of ratio, proportion, or standardization. I hope that by now you have overcome any such fear.

Appendixes
Index

Appendix A
1990 U.S. Census
Short and Long Forms

The actual U.S. Census long form includes repeated pages six and seven for up to seven family members.

FORM **D-1A**
(2-1-89)

U.S. DEPARTMENT OF COMMERCE
BUREAU OF THE CENSUS

NOTICE — Response to this inquiry **is required by law (Title 13, U.S. Code)**. By the same law, your report to the Census Bureau is **confidential**. It may be seen only by sworn Census Bureau employees and may be used only for statistical purposes.

OMB No. 0607-0628: Approval Expires 07/31/91

ENUMERATOR
QUESTIONNAIRE

1990 Census of

the United States

[short form]

COMPLETE BEFORE THE INTERVIEW

A. DO code	**B.** Unit ID	**C.** ARA	**D.** Block	**E.** Map spot	**F.** Form type	**G.** Added unit (mail-back only)
					S	1 ○ Yes 2 ○ No

H. Mailing address — Number, street, apartment number or location, rural route and box, post office box

City

State   ZIP Code

INTRODUCTIONS

- FOR MAIL-BACK AREAS (PERSONAL VISIT)

  Hello, my name is *(Your name)* **and I'm from the United States Census Bureau. This is my identification** *(PAUSE)* **and here's some information about the purpose of my visit.** *(Give respondent copy of Privacy Act Notice.)* **We are taking the 1990 census of the United States. Is this** *(Read address)***?**

  If YES — **Our records show that we have not received a census form for this address so I'm here to help you complete one. For the average household, this interview should take about 7 minutes.**

  If NO — **Can you tell me where to find** *(Read address)***?**

- FOR LIST/ENUMERATE AREAS (PERSONAL VISIT)

  Hello, my name is *(Your name)* **and I'm from the United States Census Bureau. This is my identification** *(PAUSE)* **and here's some information about the purpose of my visit.** *(Give respondent copy of Privacy Act Notice.)*

  NEXT:

  Ask the questions at the top of the listing page.

  Obtain a completed form from each address.

- FOR TELEPHONE INTERVIEW (ALL AREAS)

  Hello, my name is *(Your name)* **and I'm calling for the United States Census Bureau. Have I reached** *(Read address)***?**

  If YES — **We are taking the 1990 census of the United States and our records show that we did not receive a census form for this address. I'd like to complete the form now over the telephone. For the average household, this interview should take about 7 minutes.**

  If NO — **Excuse me. I might have dialed the wrong number. Is this** *(Read area code and phone number)***?**

COMPLETE AFTER THE INTERVIEW

I. Method of completion — *Fill ONE circle*

  1 ○ Personal visit
  2 ○ Telephone

J. Respondent's name

K. Respondent's telephone number — *Include area code*

L. Population	**M.** Vacant	**N.** Last resort	**O.** Continuation form
	1 ○ Regular	○ Yes	○ Yes
	2 ○ Usual home elsewhere		

P. CERTIFICATION — I certify that the entries I have made on this questionnaire are true and correct to the best of my knowledge.

Enumerator's signature		Date
Crew leader's initials	Date	CLD number

NOTES

The 1990 census must count every person at his or her "usual residence." This means the place where the person lives and sleeps most of the time.

Include	Do NOT include
• Everyone who usually lives here such as family members, housemates and roommates, foster children, roomers, boarders, and live-in employees	• Persons who usually live somewhere else
• Persons who are temporarily away on a business trip, on vacation, or in a general hospital	• Persons who are away in an institution such as a prison, mental hospital, or a nursing home
• College students who stay here while attending college	• College students who live somewhere else while attending college
• Persons in the Armed Forces who live here	• Persons in the Armed Forces who live somewhere else
• Newborn babies still in the hospital	
• Children in boarding schools below the college level	
• Persons who stay here most of the week while working even if they have a home somewhere else	• Persons who stay somewhere else most of the week while working
• Persons with no other home who are staying here on April 1	

1a. **Please give me the name of each person living here on Sunday, April 1, including all persons staying here who have no other home. If EVERYONE is staying here temporarily and usually lives somewhere else, give me the name of each person. Begin with the household member in whose name the home is owned, being bought, or rented. If there is no such person, start with any adult household member.**
Print last name, first name, and middle initial for each person.

	LAST	FIRST	INITIAL		LAST	FIRST	INITIAL
1				7			
2				8			
3				9			
4				10			
5				11			
6				12			

1b. *If EVERYONE listed above is staying here only temporarily and usually lives somewhere else, fill this circle* ⟶ ○
and ask — **Where do these people usually live?**
DO NOT PRINT THE ADDRESS LISTED IN ITEM H ON THE FRONT COVER.

House number	Street or road/Rural route and box number	Apartment number
City	State	ZIP Code
County or foreign country	Names of nearest intersecting streets or roads	

PLEASE ALSO ASK HOUSING QUESTIONS ON PAGE 3 →

	PERSON 1	PERSON 2	PERSON 3
Please fill one column → for each person listed in Question 1a on page 1.	Last name / First name / Middle initial	Last name / First name / Middle initial	Last name / First name / Middle initial

2. *Do not ask for Person 1.*
How is . . . related to *(Person 1)?*
Fill ONE circle for each person.

*If **Other relative** of person in column 1, fill circle and print exact relationship, such as mother-in-law, grandparent, son-in-law, niece, cousin, and so on.*

PERSON 1: START in this column with the household member (or one of the members) in whose name the home is owned, being bought, or rented.
If there is no such person, start in this column with any adult household member.

PERSON 2 / PERSON 3:
If a RELATIVE of Person 1:
- ○ Husband/wife
- ○ Natural-born or adopted son/daughter
- ○ Stepson/ stepdaughter
- ○ Brother/sister
- ○ Father/mother
- ○ Grandchild
- ○ Other relative →

If NOT RELATED to Person 1:
- ○ Roomer, boarder, or foster child
- ○ Housemate, roommate
- ○ Unmarried partner
- ○ Other nonrelative

3. Is . . . male or female?
Fill ONE circle for each person.
- ○ Male   ○ Female (each person)

4. What is . . .'s race? For example, White, Black, American Indian, Eskimo, Aleut or an Asian or Pacific Islander group such as Chinese, Filipino, Hawaiian, Korean, Vietnamese, Japanese, Asian Indian, Samoan, Guamanian, and so on.
Fill ONE circle for the race that the person considers himself/herself to be.
If response is "American Indian," ask —
What is the name of . . .'s enrolled or principal tribe?
If response is an "Other API" group such as Cambodian, Tongan, Laotian, Hmong, Thai, Pakistani, and so on, fill the "Other API" circle and print the name of the group.
If response is "Other race," ask —
Which group does . . . consider (himself/herself) to be?

Each person:
- ○ White
- ○ Black or Negro
- ○ Indian (Amer.) *(Print the name of the enrolled or principal tribe.)* →
- ○ Eskimo
- ○ Aleut

Asian or Pacific Islander (API)
- ○ Chinese   ○ Japanese
- ○ Filipino   ○ Asian Indian
- ○ Hawaiian   ○ Samoan
- ○ Korean   ○ Guamanian
- ○ Vietnamese   ○ Other API →
- ○ Other race *(Print race)* →

5. AGE AND YEAR OF BIRTH
a. How old is . . . ?
(Age should be as of April 1, 1990.)
If unknown, say —
Please give me your best estimate.
Print the age in the boxes, then fill the matching circle under each box.
b. In what year was . . . born?
Print the year of birth in the boxes, then fill the matching circle below each box.

a. Age: 0 1 2 3 4 5 6 7 8 9
b. Year of birth: 1 8 ... (tens/ones 0–9)

6. Is . . . now married, widowed, divorced, separated, or has . . . never been married?
Fill ONE circle for each person.
- ○ Now married   ○ Separated
- ○ Widowed   ○ Never married
- ○ Divorced

7. Is . . . of Spanish/Hispanic origin?
For example: Mexican, Mexican-American, Chicano, Puerto Rican, Cuban, Spaniard, or from the Spanish-speaking countries of Central or South America.
If "Yes," ask —
Which Spanish/Hispanic group is . . . ?
Fill the appropriate circle and if "Other Spanish/Hispanic," print one group.
- ○ No (not Spanish/Hispanic)
- ○ Yes, Mexican, Mexican-Am., Chicano
- ○ Yes, Puerto Rican
- ○ Yes, Cuban
- ○ Yes, other Spanish/Hispanic *(Print one group, for example: Argentinean, Colombian, Dominican, Nicaraguan, Salvadoran, Spaniard, and so on.)* →

FOR CENSUS USE →
○
○

PLEASE ALSO ASK HOUSING QUESTIONS ON PAGE 3 ——————————→

PERSON 4	PERSON 5	PERSON 6
Last name	Last name	Last name
First name — Middle initial	First name — Middle initial	First name — Middle initial

If a RELATIVE of Person 1:	If a RELATIVE of Person 1:	If a RELATIVE of Person 1:
○ Husband/wife ○ Brother/sister	○ Husband/wife ○ Brother/sister	○ Husband/wife ○ Brother/sister
○ Natural-born ○ Father/mother	○ Natural-born ○ Father/mother	○ Natural-born ○ Father/mother
or adopted ○ Grandchild	or adopted ○ Grandchild	or adopted ○ Grandchild
son/daughter ○ Other relative	son/daughter ○ Other relative	son/daughter ○ Other relative
○ Stepson/	○ Stepson/	○ Stepson/
stepdaughter	stepdaughter	stepdaughter

If NOT RELATED to Person 1:	If NOT RELATED to Person 1:	If NOT RELATED to Person 1:
○ Roomer, boarder, ○ Unmarried	○ Roomer, boarder, ○ Unmarried	○ Roomer, boarder, ○ Unmarried
or foster child partner	or foster child partner	or foster child partner
○ Housemate, ■ ○ Other	○ Housemate, ■ ○ Other	○ Housemate, ■ ○ Other
roommate nonrelative	roommate nonrelative	roommate nonrelative

○ Male ○ Female	○ Male ○ Female	○ Male ○ Female

○ White	○ White	○ White
○ Black or Negro	○ Black or Negro	○ Black or Negro
○ Indian (Amer.) *(Print the name of the enrolled or principal tribe.)*	○ Indian (Amer.) *(Print the name of the enrolled or principal tribe.)*	○ Indian (Amer.) *(Print the name of the enrolled or principal tribe.)*
○ Eskimo	○ Eskimo	○ Eskimo
○ Aleut Asian or Pacific Islander (API)	○ Aleut Asian or Pacific Islander (API)	○ Aleut Asian or Pacific Islander (API)
○ Chinese ○ Japanese	○ Chinese ○ Japanese	○ Chinese ○ Japanese
○ Filipino ■ ○ Asian Indian	○ Filipino ■ ○ Asian Indian	○ Filipino ■ ○ Asian Indian
○ Hawaiian ○ Samoan	○ Hawaiian ○ Samoan	○ Hawaiian ○ Samoan
○ Korean ○ Guamanian	○ Korean ○ Guamanian	○ Korean ○ Guamanian
○ Vietnamese ○ Other API	○ Vietnamese ○ Other API	○ Vietnamese ○ Other API
○ Other race *(Print race)*	○ Other race *(Print race)*	○ Other race *(Print race)*

a. Age	b. Year of birth	a. Age	b. Year of birth	a. Age	b. Year of birth
0 0 0 0 0	1●8 0 0 0 0	0 0 0 0 0	1●8 0 0 0 0	0 0 0 0 0	1●8 0 0 0 0
1 0 1 0 1 0	9 0 1 0 1 0	1 0 1 0 1 0	9 0 1 0 1 0	1 0 1 0 1 0	9 0 1 0 1 0
2 0 2 0	2 0 2 0	2 0 2 0	2 0 2 0	2 0 2 0	2 0 2 0
3 0 3 0	3 0 3 0	3 0 3 0	3 0 3 0	3 0 3 0	3 0 3 0
4 0 4 0 ■	4 0 4 0	4 0 4 0 ■	4 0 4 0	4 0 4 0 ■	4 0 4 0
5 0 5 0	5 0 5 0	5 0 5 0	5 0 5 0	5 0 5 0	5 0 5 0
6 0 6 0	6 0 6 0	6 0 6 0	6 0 6 0	6 0 6 0	6 0 6 0
7 0 7 0	7 0 7 0	7 0 7 0	7 0 7 0	7 0 7 0	7 0 7 0
8 0 8 0	8 0 8 0	8 0 8 0	8 0 8 0	8 0 8 0	8 0 8 0
9 0 9 0	9 0 9 0	9 0 9 0	9 0 9 0	9 0 9 0	9 0 9 0

○ Now married ○ Separated	○ Now married ○ Separated	○ Now married ○ Separated
○ Widowed ○ Never married	○ Widowed ○ Never married	○ Widowed ○ Never married
○ Divorced	○ Divorced	○ Divorced

○ No (not Spanish/Hispanic)	○ No (not Spanish/Hispanic)	○ No (not Spanish/Hispanic)
○ Yes, Mexican, Mexican-Am., Chicano	○ Yes, Mexican, Mexican-Am., Chicano	○ Yes, Mexican, Mexican-Am., Chicano
○ Yes, Puerto Rican ■	○ Yes, Puerto Rican ■	○ Yes, Puerto Rican
○ Yes, Cuban	○ Yes, Cuban	○ Yes, Cuban
○ Yes, other Spanish/Hispanic	○ Yes, other Spanish/Hispanic	○ Yes, other Spanish/Hispanic
(Print one group, for example: Argentinean, Colombian, Dominican, Nicaraguan, Salvadoran, Spaniard, and so on.)	*(Print one group, for example: Argentinean, Colombian, Dominican, Nicaraguan, Salvadoran, Spaniard, and so on.)*	*(Print one group, for example: Argentinean, Colombian, Dominican, Nicaraguan, Salvadoran, Spaniard, and so on.)*

○	○	○
○	○	○

PERSON 7

Last name

First name / **Middle initial**

If a RELATIVE of Person 1:
- ○ Husband/wife ○ Brother/sister
- ○ Natural-born ○ Father/mother
  or adopted ○ Grandchild
  son/daughter ○ Other relative ⌐7
- ○ Stepson/
  stepdaughter [   ]

If NOT RELATED to Person 1:
- ○ Roomer, boarder, ○ Unmarried
  or foster child partner
- ○ Housemate, ○ Other
  roommate nonrelative

- ○ Male ○ Female

- ○ White
- ○ Black or Negro
- ○ Indian (Amer.) *(Print the name of the enrolled or principal tribe.)* ⌐7
  [   ]
- ○ Eskimo
- ○ Aleut

Asian or Pacific Islander (API)
- ○ Chinese ○ Japanese
- ○ Filipino ○ Asian Indian
- ○ Hawaiian ○ Samoan
- ○ Korean ○ Guamanian
- ○ Vietnamese ○ Other API ⌐7
  [   ]
- ○ Other race *(Print race)* ⌐⌐

a. Age	b. Year of birth
[ ]	*1* [ ]

0	0	0	0	0	0	1 ●	8	0	0	0	0
1	0	1	0	1	0	9	0	1	0	1	0
2	0	2	0			2	0	2	0		
3	0	3	0			3	0	3	0		
4	0	4	0			4	0	4	0		
5	0	5	0			5	0	5	0		
6	0	6	0			6	0	6	0		
7	0	7	0			7	0	7	0		
8	0	8	0			8	0	8	0		
9	0	9	0			9	0	9	0		

- ○ Now married ○ Separated
- ○ Widowed ○ Never married
- ○ Divorced

- ○ No (not Spanish/Hispanic)
- ○ Yes, Mexican, Mexican-Am., Chicano
- ○ Yes, Puerto Rican
- ○ Yes, Cuban
- ○ Yes, other Spanish/Hispanic
  (Print one group, for example: Argentinean, Colombian, Dominican, Nicaraguan, Salvadoran, Spaniard, and so on.) ⌐7
  [   ]

- ○
- ○

H1a. When you told me the names of persons living here on April 1, did you leave anyone out because you were not sure if the person should be listed — for example, someone temporarily away on a business trip or vacation, a newborn baby still in the hospital, or a person who stays here once in a while and has no other home?
- ○ Yes — *Determine if you should add the person(s) based on the instructions for Question 1a.* ○ No

b. When you told me the names of persons living here on April 1, did you include anyone even though you were not sure that the person should be listed — for example, a visitor who is staying here temporarily or a person who usually lives somewhere else?
- ○ Yes — *Determine if you should delete the person(s) based on the instructions for Question 1a.* ○ No

H2. Which best describes this building? Include all apartments, flats, etc., even if vacant.
- ○ A mobile home or trailer
- ○ A one-family house detached from any other house
- ○ A one-family house attached to one or more houses
- ○ A building with 2 apartments
- ○ A building with 3 or 4 apartments
- ○ A building with 5 to 9 apartments
- ○ A building with 10 to 19 apartments
- ○ A building with 20 to 49 apartments
- ○ A building with 50 or more apartments
- ○ Other

H3. How many rooms do you have in this (house/apartment)? Do NOT count bathrooms, porches, balconies, foyers, halls, or half-rooms.
- ○ 1 room ○ 4 rooms ○ 7 rooms
- ○ 2 rooms ○ 5 rooms ○ 8 rooms
- ○ 3 rooms ○ 6 rooms ○ 9 or more rooms

H4. Is this (house/apartment) —
- ○ Owned by you or someone in this household with a mortgage or loan?
- ○ Owned by you or someone in this household free and clear (without a mortgage)?
- ○ Rented for cash rent?
- ○ Occupied without payment of cash rent?

If this is a ONE-FAMILY HOUSE —
H5a. Is this house on ten or more acres?
- ○ Yes ○ No

b. is there a business (such as a store or barber shop) or a medical office on this property?
- ○ Yes ○ No

Ask only if someone in this household OWNS OR IS BUYING this house or apartment —
H6. What is the value of this property; that is, how much do you think this (house and lot/condominium unit) would sell for if it were for sale?

○ Less than $10,000	○ $70,000 to $74,999
○ $10,000 to $14,999	○ $75,000 to $79,999
○ $15,000 to $19,999	○ $80,000 to $89,999
○ $20,000 to $24,999	○ $90,000 to $99,999
○ $25,000 to $29,999	○ $100,000 to $124,999
○ $30,000 to $34,999	○ $125,000 to $149,999
○ $35,000 to $39,999	○ $150,000 to $174,999
○ $40,000 to $44,999	○ $175,000 to $199,999
○ $45,000 to $49,999	○ $200,000 to $249,999
○ $50,000 to $54,999	○ $250,000 to $299,999
○ $55,000 to $59,999	○ $300,000 to $399,999
○ $60,000 to $64,999	○ $400,000 to $499,999
○ $65,000 to $69,999	○ $500,000 or more

Ask only if RENT IS PAID for this house or apartment —
H7a. What is the monthly rent?
If rent is NOT PAID BY THE MONTH, see your job instructions on how to figure a monthly rent.

○ Less than $80	○ $375 to $399
○ $80 to $99	○ $400 to $424
○ $100 to $124	○ $425 to $449
○ $125 to $149	○ $450 to $474
○ $150 to $174	○ $475 to $499
○ $175 to $199	○ $500 to $524
○ $200 to $224	○ $525 to $549
○ $225 to $249	○ $550 to $599
○ $250 to $274	○ $600 to $649
○ $275 to $299	○ $650 to $699
○ $300 to $324	○ $700 to $749
○ $325 to $349	○ $750 to $999
○ $350 to $374	○ $1,000 or more

b. Does the monthly rent include any meals?
- ○ Yes ○ No

FOR CENSUS USE					

A. Total persons [   ]

B. Type of unit

	Occupied	Vacant
○ First form	○ Regular	
○ Cont'n	○ Usual home elsewhere	

0	0
1	1
2	2
	3
	4
	5
	6
	7
	8
	9

C1. Vacancy status
- ○ For rent ○ For seas/ rec/occ
- ○ For sale only
- ○ Rented or sold, not occupied ○ For migrant workers ○ Other vacant

C2. Is this unit boarded up?
- ○ Yes ○ No

D. Months vacant
- ○ Less than 1 ○ 6 up to 12
- ○ 1 up to 2 ○ 12 up to 24
- ○ 2 up to 6 ○ 24 or more

E. Complete after
- ○ LR ○ TC ○ QA JIC 1
- ○ P/F ○ RE ○ I/T
- ○ MV ○ ED ○ EN

- ○ P0 ○ P3 ○ P6
- ○ P1 ○ P4 ○ IA JIC 2
- ○ P2 ○ P5 ○ SM ○

F. Cov.
- ○ 1b ○ 1a ○ 7 ○ H1

G. DO **ID**

0	0	0	0	0	0	0	0	0	0
1	1	1	1	1	1	1	1	1	1
2	2	2	2	2	2	2	2	2	2
3	3	3	3	3	3	3	3	3	3
4	4	4	4	4	4	4	4	4	4
5	5	5	5	5	5	5	5	5	5
6	6	6	6	6	6	6	6	6	6
7	7	7	7	7	7	7	7	7	7
8	8	8	8	8	8	8	8	8	8
9	9	9	9	9	9	9	9	9	9

OMB No. 0607-0628: Approval Expires 07/31/91

| FORM **D-2A** (2-1-89) | U.S. DEPARTMENT OF COMMERCE BUREAU OF THE CENSUS | NOTICE — Response to this inquiry **is required by law (Title 13, U.S. Code)**. By the same law, your report to the Census Bureau is **confidential**. It may be seen only by sworn Census Bureau employees and may be used only for statistical purposes. |

ENUMERATOR QUESTIONNAIRE

1990 Census of the United States

[long form]

COMPLETE BEFORE THE INTERVIEW

A. DO code	**B.** Unit ID	**C.** ARA	**D.** Block	**E.** Map spot	**F.** Form type	**G.** Added unit (mail-back only)
					L	1 ○ Yes 2 ○ No

H. Mailing address — Number, street, apartment number or location, rural route and box, post office box

City

State   ZIP Code

INTRODUCTIONS

- **FOR MAIL-BACK AREAS (PERSONAL VISIT)**

Hello, my name is *(Your name)* **and I'm from the United States Census Bureau. This is my identification** *(PAUSE)* **and here's some information about the purpose of my visit.** *(Give respondent copy of Privacy Act Notice.)* **We are taking the 1990 census of the United States. Is this** *(Read address)***?**

  If YES — **Our records show that we have not received a census form for this address so I'm here to help you complete one. For the average household, this interview should take about 26 minutes.**

  If NO — **Can you tell me where to find** *(Read address)***?**

- **FOR LIST/ENUMERATE AREAS (PERSONAL VISIT)**

Hello, my name is *(Your name)* **and I'm from the United States Census Bureau. This is my identification** *(PAUSE)* **and here's some information about the purpose of my visit.** *(Give respondent copy of Privacy Act Notice.)*

  NEXT:

  Ask the questions at the top of the listing page.

  Obtain a completed form from each address.

- **FOR TELEPHONE INTERVIEW (ALL AREAS)**

Hello, my name is *(Your name)* **and I'm calling for the United States Census Bureau. Have I reached** *(Read address)***?**

  If YES — **We are taking the 1990 census of the United States and our records show that we did not receive a census form for this address. I'd like to complete the form now over the telephone. For the average household, this interview should take about 26 minutes.**

  If NO — **Excuse me. I might have dialed the wrong number. Is this** *(Read area code and phone number)***?**

COMPLETE AFTER THE INTERVIEW

I. Method of completion — *Fill ONE circle*

1 ○ Personal visit

2 ○ Telephone

J. Respondent's name

K. Respondent's telephone number — *Include area code*

L. Population	**M.** Vacant	**N.** Last resort	**O.** Continuation form
	1 ○ Regular	○ Yes	○ Yes
	2 ○ Usual home elsewhere		

P. CERTIFICATION — I certify that the entries I have made on this questionnaire are true and correct to the best of my knowledge.

Enumerator's signature		Date
Crew leader's initials	Date	CLD number

NOTES

The 1990 census must count every person at his or her "usual residence." This means the place where the person lives and sleeps most of the time.

Include

- Everyone who usually lives here such as family members, housemates and roommates, foster children, roomers, boarders, and live-in employees
- Persons who are temporarily away on a business trip, on vacation, or in a general hospital
- College students who stay here while attending college
- Persons in the Armed Forces who live here
- Newborn babies still in the hospital
- Children in boarding schools below the college level
- Persons who stay here most of the week while working even if they have a home somewhere else
- Persons with no other home who are staying here on April 1

Do NOT include

- Persons who usually live somewhere else
- Persons who are away in an institution such as a prison, mental hospital, or a nursing home
- College students who live somewhere else while attending college
- Persons in the Armed Forces who live somewhere else
- Persons who stay somewhere else most of the week while working

1a. **Please give me the name of each person living here on Sunday, April 1, including all persons staying here who have no other home. If EVERYONE is staying here temporarily and usually lives somewhere else, give me the name of each person. Begin with the household member in whose name the home is owned, being bought, or rented. If there is no such person, start with any adult household member.**
Print last name, first name, and middle initial for each person.

	LAST	FIRST	INITIAL		LAST	FIRST	INITIAL
1				7			
2				8			
3				9			
4				10			
5				11			
6				12			

1b. *If EVERYONE listed above is staying here only temporarily and usually lives somewhere else, fill this circle* ⟶ ○
and ask — **Where do these people usually live?**
DO NOT PRINT THE ADDRESS LISTED IN ITEM H ON THE FRONT COVER.

House number	Street or road/Rural route and box number	Apartment number

City	State	ZIP Code

County or foreign country	Names of nearest intersecting streets or roads

PLEASE ALSO ASK HOUSING QUESTIONS

	PERSON 1	PERSON 2
Please fill one column → for each person listed in Question 1a on page 1.	Last name First name — Middle initial	Last name First name — Middle initial

2. *Do not ask for Person 1.*
How is . . . related to *(Person 1)?*
Fill ONE circle for each person.

If **Other relative** *of person in column 1, fill circle and print exact relationship, such as mother-in-law, grandparent, son-in-law, niece, cousin, and so on.*

PERSON 1:
START in this column with the household member (or one of the members) in whose name the home is owned, being bought, or rented.

If there is no such person, start in this column with any adult household member.

■

PERSON 2:
If a RELATIVE of Person 1:
- ○ Husband/wife   ○ Brother/sister
- ○ Natural-born   ○ Father/mother
  or adopted   ○ Grandchild
  son/daughter   ○ Other relative ⌐
- ○ Stepson/
  stepdaughter   [_____]

If NOT RELATED to Person 1:
- ○ Roomer, boarder,   ○ Unmarried
  or foster child   partner
- ○ Housemate, ■   ○ Other
  roommate   nonrelative

3. Is . . . male or female?
Fill ONE circle for each person.

PERSON 1: ○ Male   ○ Female
PERSON 2: ○ Male   ○ Female

4. What is . . .'s race? For example, White, Black, American Indian, Eskimo, Aleut or an Asian or Pacific Islander group such as Chinese, Filipino, Hawaiian, Korean, Vietnamese, Japanese, Asian Indian, Samoan, Guamanian, and so on.
Fill ONE circle for the race that the person considers himself/herself to be.
If response is "American Indian," ask —
What is the name of . . .'s enrolled or principal tribe?
If response is an "Other API" group such as Cambodian, Tongan, Laotian, Hmong, Thai, Pakistani, and so on, fill the "Other API" circle and print the name of the group.
If response is "Other race," ask —
Which group does . . . consider (himself/herself) to be?

PERSON 1:
- ○ White
- ○ Black or Negro
- ○ Indian (Amer.) *(Print the name of the enrolled or principal tribe.)* ⌐
  [_____]
- ○ Eskimo
- ○ Aleut   Asian or Pacific Islander (API)
- ○ Chinese ■   ○ Japanese
- ○ Filipino   ○ Asian Indian
- ○ Hawaiian   ○ Samoan
- ○ Korean   ○ Guamanian
- ○ Vietnamese   ○ Other API ⌐
  [_____]
- ○ Other race *(Print race)* ⌐

PERSON 2:
- ○ White
- ○ Black or Negro
- ○ Indian (Amer.) *(Print the name of the enrolled or principal tribe.)* ⌐
  [_____]
- ○ Eskimo
- ○ Aleut   Asian or Pacific Islander (API)
- ○ Chinese ■   ○ Japanese
- ○ Filipino   ○ Asian Indian
- ○ Hawaiian   ○ Samoan
- ○ Korean   ○ Guamanian
- ○ Vietnamese   ○ Other API ⌐
  [_____]
- ○ Other race *(Print race)* ⌐

5. AGE AND YEAR OF BIRTH

a. How old is . . . ?
(Age should be as of April 1, 1990.)

If unknown, say —
Please give me your best estimate.
Print the age in the boxes, then fill the matching circle under each box.

b. In what year was . . . born?
Print the year of birth in the boxes, then fill the matching circle below each box.

PERSON 1:
a. Age [| | |]
0 0 0 0 0
1 ○ 1 0 1 0
2 0 2 0
3 ○ 3 0
4 0 4 0 ■
5 0 5 0
6 0 6 0
7 0 7 0
8 0 8 0
9 0 9 0

b. Year of birth *1* [| | |]
1 ● 8 0 0 0 0
9 0 1 0 1 0
2 0 2 0
3 0 3 0
4 0 4 0
5 0 5 0
6 0 6 0
7 0 7 0
8 0 8 0
9 0 9 0

PERSON 2:
a. Age [| | |]
0 0 0 0 0
1 ○ 1 0 1 0
2 0 2 0
3 0 3 0
4 0 4 0 ■
5 0 5 0
6 0 6 0
7 0 7 0
8 0 8 0
9 0 9 0

b. Year of birth *1* [| | |]
1 ● 8 0 0 0 0
9 0 1 0 1 0
2 0 2 0
3 0 3 0
4 0 4 0
5 0 5 0
6 0 6 0
7 0 7 0
8 0 8 0
9 0 9 0

6. Is . . . now married, widowed, divorced, separated, or has . . . never been married?
Fill ONE circle for each person.

PERSON 1:
- ○ Now married   ○ Separated
- ○ Widowed   ○ Never married
- ○ Divorced

PERSON 2:
- ○ Now married   ○ Separated
- ○ Widowed   ○ Never married
- ○ Divorced

7. Is . . . of Spanish/Hispanic origin?
For example: Mexican, Mexican-American, Chicano, Puerto Rican, Cuban, Spaniard, or from the Spanish-speaking countries of Central or South America.

If "Yes," ask —
Which Spanish/Hispanic group is . . . ?
Fill the appropriate circle and if "Other Spanish/Hispanic," print one group.

PERSON 1:
- ○ No (not Spanish/Hispanic)
- ○ Yes, Mexican, Mexican-Am., Chicano
- ○ Yes, Puerto Rican ■
- ○ Yes, Cuban
- ○ Yes, other Spanish/Hispanic
  (Print one group, for example: Argentinean, Colombian, Dominican, Nicaraguan, Salvadoran, Spaniard, and so on.) ⌐
  [_____]

PERSON 2:
- ○ No (not Spanish/Hispanic)
- ○ Yes, Mexican, Mexican-Am., Chicano
- ○ Yes, Puerto Rican
- ○ Yes, Cuban
- ○ Yes, other Spanish/Hispanic
  (Print one group, for example: Argentinean, Colombian, Dominican, Nicaraguan, Salvadoran, Spaniard, and so on.) ⌐
  [_____]

FOR CENSUS USE →

PERSON 1: ○ ○
PERSON 2: ○ ○

S ON PAGE 3 ⟶   PLEASE ALSO ASK HOUSING QUESTIONS ON PAGE 3 ⟶

PERSON 3	PERSON 4	PERSON 5	PERSON 6
Last name	Last name	Last name	Last name
First name Middle initial	First name Middle initial	First name Middle initial	First name Middle initial

If a RELATIVE of Person 1: (all four columns identical)
- ○ Husband/wife
- ○ Natural-born or adopted son/daughter
- ○ Stepson/stepdaughter
- ○ Brother/sister
- ○ Father/mother
- ○ Grandchild
- ○ Other relative ⌐

If NOT RELATED to Person 1: (all four columns identical)
- ○ Roomer, boarder, or foster child
- ○ Housemate, roommate ■
- ○ Unmarried partner
- ○ Other nonrelative

- ○ Male   ○ Female

Race (all four columns identical):
- ○ White
- ○ Black or Negro
- ○ Indian (Amer.) *(Print the name of the enrolled or principal tribe.)* ⌐
- ○ Eskimo
- ○ Aleut

Asian or Pacific Islander (API)
- ○ Chinese   ■   ○ Japanese
- ○ Filipino   ○ Asian Indian
- ○ Hawaiian   ○ Samoan
- ○ Korean   ○ Guamanian
- ○ Vietnamese   ○ Other API ⌐

- ○ Other race *(Print race)* ⌐

(For Persons 3, 5, 6 the ■ appears at Filipino row; for Person 4 ■ appears at Chinese row)

a. Age   **b. Year of birth** (all four columns identical)

a. Age	b. Year of birth
0 ○ 0 ○ 0 ○	1 ● 8 ○ 0 ○ 0 ○
1 ○ 1 ○ 1 ○	9 ○ 1 ○ 1 ○
2 ○ 2 ○	2 ○ 2 ○
3 ○ 3 ○	3 ○ 3 ○
4 ○ 4 ○	4 ○ 4 ○
5 ○ 5 ○	5 ○ 5 ○
6 ○ 6 ○	6 ○ 6 ○
7 ○ 7 ○	7 ○ 7 ○
8 ○ 8 ○	8 ○ 8 ○
9 ○ 9 ○	9 ○ 9 ○

Marital status (all four columns identical):
- ○ Now married   ○ Separated
- ○ Widowed   ○ Never married
- ○ Divorced

Hispanic origin (all four columns identical):
- ○ No (not Spanish/Hispanic)
- ○ Yes, Mexican, Mexican-Am., Chicano
- ○ Yes, Puerto Rican ■
- ○ Yes, Cuban
- ○ Yes, other Spanish/Hispanic *(Print one group, for example: Argentinean, Colombian, Dominican, Nicaraguan, Salvadoran, Spaniard, and so on.)* ⌐

- ○
- ○

PERSON 7

Last name

First name   Middle initial

If a RELATIVE of Person 1:

- ○ Husband/wife
- ○ Natural-born or adopted son/daughter
- ○ Stepson/ stepdaughter
- ○ Brother/sister
- ○ Father/mother
- ○ Grandchild
- ○ Other relative ⌐

If NOT RELATED to Person 1:

- ○ Roomer, boarder, or foster child
- ○ Housemate, roommate
- ○ Unmarried partner
- ○ Other nonrelative

- ○ Male
- ○ Female

- ○ White
- ○ Black or Negro
- ○ Indian (Amer.) *(Print the name of the enrolled or principal tribe.)* ⌐
- ○ Eskimo
- ○ Aleut

Asian or Pacific Islander (API)

- ○ Chinese
- ○ Filipino
- ○ Hawaiian
- ○ Korean
- ○ Vietnamese
- ○ Japanese
- ○ Asian Indian
- ○ Samoan
- ○ Guamanian
- ○ Other API ⌐

- ○ Other race *(Print race)* ⌐

a. Age | b. Year of birth

1

0	0	0	0	0		1 ●	8	0	0	0	0
1	0	1	0	1	0		9	0	1	0	1	0
2		2	0	2	0			2	0	2	0
3	0	3	0				3	0	3	0
4	0	4	0				4	0	4	0
5	0	5	0				5	0	5	0
6	0	6	0				6	0	6	0
7	0	7	0				7	0	7	0
8	0	8	0				8	0	8	0
9	0	9	0				9	0	9	0

- ○ Now married
- ○ Widowed
- ○ Divorced
- ○ Separated
- ○ Never married

- ○ No (not Spanish/Hispanic)
- ○ Yes, Mexican, Mexican-Am., Chicano
- ○ Yes, Puerto Rican
- ○ Yes, Cuban
- ○ Yes, other Spanish/Hispanic *(Print one group, for example: Argentinean, Colombian, Dominican, Nicaraguan, Salvadoran, Spaniard, and so on.)* ⌐

- ○
- ○

H1a. When you told me the names of persons living here on April 1, did you leave anyone out because you were not sure if the person should be listed — for example, someone temporarily away on a business trip or vacation, a newborn baby still in the hospital, or a person who stays here once in a while and has no other home?

- ○ Yes — *Determine if you should add the person(s) based on the instructions for Question 1a.*
- ○ No

b. When you told me the names of persons living here on April 1, did you include anyone even though you were not sure that the person should be listed — for example, a visitor who is staying here temporarily or a person who usually lives somewhere else?

- ○ Yes — *Determine if you should delete the person(s) based on the instructions for Question 1a.*
- ○ No

H2. Which best describes this building? Include all apartments, flats, etc., even if vacant.

- ○ A mobile home or trailer
- ○ A one-family house detached from any other house
- ○ A one-family house attached to one or more houses
- ○ A building with 2 apartments
- ○ A building with 3 or 4 apartments
- ○ A building with 5 to 9 apartments
- ○ A building with 10 to 19 apartments
- ○ A building with 20 to 49 apartments
- ○ A building with 50 or more apartments
- ○ Other

H3. How many rooms do you have in this (house/apartment)? Do NOT count bathrooms, porches, balconies, foyers, halls, or half-rooms.

- ○ 1 room
- ○ 2 rooms
- ○ 3 rooms
- ○ 4 rooms
- ○ 5 rooms
- ○ 6 rooms
- ○ 7 rooms
- ○ 8 rooms
- ○ 9 or more rooms

H4. Is this (house/apartment) —

- ○ Owned by you or someone in this household with a mortgage or loan?
- ○ Owned by you or someone in this household free and clear (without a mortgage)?
- ○ Rented for cash rent?
- ○ Occupied without payment of cash rent?

If this is a ONE-FAMILY HOUSE —

H5a. Is this house on ten or more acres?

- ○ Yes
- ○ No

b. Is there a business (such as a store or barber shop) or a medical office on this property?

- ○ Yes
- ○ No

Ask only if someone in this household OWNS OR IS BUYING this house or apartment —

H6. What is the value of this property; that is, how much do you think this (house and lot/condominium unit) would sell for if it were for sale?

○ Less than $10,000	○ $70,000 to $74,999
○ $10,000 to $14,999	○ $75,000 to $79,999
○ $15,000 to $19,999	○ $80,000 to $89,999
○ $20,000 to $24,999	○ $90,000 to $99,999
○ $25,000 to $29,999	○ $100,000 to $124,999
○ $30,000 to $34,999	○ $125,000 to $149,999
○ $35,000 to $39,999	○ $150,000 to $174,999
○ $40,000 to $44,999	○ $175,000 to $199,999
○ $45,000 to $49,999	○ $200,000 to $249,999
○ $50,000 to $54,999	○ $250,000 to $299,999
○ $55,000 to $59,999	○ $300,000 to $399,999
○ $60,000 to $64,999	○ $400,000 to $499,999
○ $65,000 to $69,999	○ $500,000 or more

Ask only if RENT IS PAID for this house or apartment —

H7a. What is the monthly rent?
If rent is NOT PAID BY THE MONTH, see your job instructions on how to figure a monthly rent.

○ Less than $80	○ $375 to $399
○ $80 to $99	○ $400 to $424
○ $100 to $124	○ $425 to $449
○ $125 to $149	○ $450 to $474
○ $150 to $174	○ $475 to $499
○ $175 to $199	○ $500 to $524
○ $200 to $224	○ $525 to $549
○ $225 to $249	○ $550 to $599
○ $250 to $274	○ $600 to $649
○ $275 to $299	○ $650 to $699
○ $300 to $324	○ $700 to $749
○ $325 to $349	○ $750 to $999
○ $350 to $374	○ $1,000 or more

b. Does the monthly rent include any meals?

- ○ Yes
- ○ No

FOR CENSUS USE

A. Total persons

B. Type of unit

Occupied	Vacant
○ First form	○ Regular
○ Cont'n	○ Usual home elsewhere

C1. Vacancy status

- ○ For rent
- ○ For sale only
- ○ Rented or sold, not occupied
- ○ For seas/ rec/occ
- ○ For migrant workers
- ○ Other vacant

C2. Is this unit boarded up?

- ○ Yes
- ○ No

D. Months vacant

- ○ Less than 1
- ○ 1 up to 2
- ○ 2 up to 6
- ○ 6 up to 12
- ○ 12 up to 24
- ○ 24 or more

E. Complete after

- ○ LR ○ TC ○ QA   JIC 1
- ○ P/F ○ RE ○ I/T
- ○ MV ○ ED ○ EN
- ○ PO ○ P3 ○ P6
- ○ P1 ○ P4 ○ IA   JIC 2
- ○ P2 ○ P5 ○ SM

F. Cov.

- ○ 1b ○ 1a ○ 7 ○ H1

G. DO   **ID**

H8. When did *(Person listed in column 1 on page 2)* move into this (house/apartment)?

- ○ 1989 or 1990
- ○ 1985 to 1988
- ○ 1980 to 1984
- ○ 1970 to 1979
- ○ 1960 to 1969
- ○ 1959 or earlier

H9. How many bedrooms do you have; that is, how many bedrooms would you list if this (house/apartment) were on the market for sale or rent?

- ○ No bedroom
- ○ 1 bedroom
- ○ 2 bedrooms
- ○ 3 bedrooms
- ○ 4 bedrooms
- ○ 5 or more bedrooms

H10. Do you have COMPLETE plumbing facilities in this (house/apartment); that is, hot and cold piped water, a flush toilet, and a bathtub or shower?

- ○ Yes, have all three facilities
- ○ No

H11. Do you have COMPLETE kitchen facilities; that is, a sink with piped water, a range or cookstove, and a refrigerator?

- ○ Yes
- ○ No

H12. Do you have a telephone in this (house/apartment)?

- ○ Yes
- ○ No

H13. How many automobiles, vans, and trucks of one-ton capacity or less are kept at home for use by members of your household?

- ○ None
- ○ 1
- ○ 2
- ○ 3
- ○ 4
- ○ 5
- ○ 6
- ○ 7 or more

H14. Which FUEL is used MOST for heating this (house/apartment)?

- ○ Gas: from underground pipes serving the neighborhood
- ○ Gas: bottled, tank, or LP
- ○ Electricity
- ○ Fuel oil, kerosene, etc.
- ○ Coal or coke
- ○ Wood
- ○ Solar energy
- ○ Other fuel
- ○ No fuel used

H15. Do you get water from —

- ○ A public system such as a city water department, or private company?
- ○ An individual drilled well?
- ○ An individual dug well?
- ○ Some other source such as a spring, creek, river, cistern, etc.?

H16. Is this building connected to a public sewer?

- ○ Yes, connected to public sewer
- ○ No, connected to septic tank or cesspool
- ○ No, use other means

H17. About when was this building first built?

- ○ 1989 or 1990
- ○ 1985 to 1988
- ○ 1980 to 1984
- ○ 1970 to 1979
- ○ 1960 to 1969
- ○ 1950 to 1959
- ○ 1940 to 1949
- ○ 1939 or earlier
- ○ Don't know

H18. Is this (house/apartment) part of a condominium?

- ○ Yes
- ○ No

If respondent reported living in an apartment building, skip to H20.

H19a. Is this house on less than 1 acre?

- ○ Yes — *Skip to H20*
- ○ No

b. In 1989, what were the actual sales of all agricultural products from this property?

- ○ None
- ○ $1 to $999
- ○ $1,000 to $2,499
- ○ $2,500 to $4,999
- ○ $5,000 to $9,999
- ○ $10,000 or more

H20. What are the yearly costs of utilities and fuels for this (house/apartment)?
If the respondent has lived here less than 1 year, obtain an estimate of yearly costs.

a. For electricity

$_____.00
Yearly cost — Dollars

OR

- ○ Included in rent or in condominium fee
- ○ No charge or electricity not used

b. For gas

$_____.00
Yearly cost — Dollars

OR

- ○ Included in rent or in condominium fee
- ○ No charge or gas not used

c. For water

$_____.00
Yearly cost — Dollars

OR

- ○ Included in rent or in condominium fee
- ○ No charge

d. For oil, coal, kerosene, wood, etc.

$_____.00
Yearly cost — Dollars

OR

- ○ Included in rent or in condominium fee
- ○ No charge or these fuels not used

INTERVIEWER INSTRUCTION:

Ask questions H21 TO H26 if this is a one-family house, a condominium, or a mobile home that someone in this household OWNS OR IS BUYING; otherwise, go to page 6.

H21. What were the real estate taxes on THIS property last year?

$ _____.00
Yearly amount — Dollars

OR

○ None

H22. What was the annual payment for fire, hazard, and flood insurance on THIS property?

$ _____.00
Yearly amount — Dollars

OR

○ None

H23a. Do you have a mortgage, deed of trust, contract to purchase, or similar debt on THIS property?

○ Yes, mortgage, deed of trust, or similar debt

○ Yes, contract to purchase } *Go to H23b*

○ No — *Skip to H24a*

b. How much is your regular monthly mortgage payment on THIS property? Include payment only on first mortgage or contract to purchase.

$ _____.00
Monthly amount — Dollars

OR

○ No regular payment required — *Skip to H24a*

c. Does your regular monthly mortgage payment include payments for real estate taxes on THIS property?

○ Yes, taxes included in payment

○ No, taxes paid separately or taxes not required

d. Does your regular monthly mortgage payment include payments for fire, hazard, or flood insurance on THIS property?

○ Yes, insurance included in payment

○ No, insurance paid separately or no insurance

H24a. Do you have a second or junior mortgage or a home equity loan on THIS property?

○ Yes

○ No — *Skip to H25*

b. How much is your regular monthly payment on all second or junior mortgages and all home equity loans?

$ _____.00
Monthly amount — Dollars

OR

○ No regular payment required

Ask ONLY if this is a CONDOMINIUM —

H25. What is the monthly condominium fee?

$ _____.00
Monthly amount — Dollars

Ask ONLY if this is a MOBILE HOME —

H26. What was the total cost for personal property taxes, site rent, registration fees, and license fees on this mobile home and its site last year? Exclude real estate taxes.

$ _____.00
Yearly amount — Dollars

Please turn to page 6. ➔

PERSON 1

Last name _____ First name _____ Middle initial

8. In what U.S. State or foreign country was . . . born?
Print the name of State or foreign country; or Puerto Rico, Guam, etc. in the space below.

9. *If the answer to question 8 appears in one of the first two "Yes" categories listed below, fill the appropriate "Yes" category. Otherwise, ask —*
Is . . . a CITIZEN of the United States? That is, does . . . have at least one American parent or is . . . a citizen by naturalization?

○ Yes, born in the United States — *Skip to 11*
○ Yes, born in Puerto Rico, Guam, the
   U.S. Virgin Islands, or Northern Marianas
○ Yes, born abroad of American parent or parents
○ Yes, U.S. citizen by naturalization
○ No, not a citizen of the United States

10. When did . . . come to the United States to stay? *If entered country more than once, ask — What is the latest year?*

○ 1987 to 1990   ■ ○ 1970 to 1974
○ 1985 or 1986   ○ 1965 to 1969
○ 1982 to 1984   ○ 1960 to 1964
○ 1980 or 1981   ○ 1950 to 1959
○ 1975 to 1979   ○ Before 1950

11. At any time since February 1, 1990, has . . . attended regular school or college? Include only nursery school, kindergarten, elementary school, and schooling which leads to a high school diploma or a college degree.
If "Yes," ask — Public or private?

○ No, has not attended since February 1
○ Yes, public school, public college
○ Yes, private school, private college

12. How much school has . . . COMPLETED?
Read categories if person is unsure. Fill ONE circle for the highest level completed or degree received. If currently enrolled, mark the level of previous grade attended or highest degree received.

○ No school completed
○ Nursery school
○ Kindergarten   ■
○ 1st, 2nd, 3rd, or 4th grade
○ 5th, 6th, 7th, or 8th grade
○ 9th grade
○ 10th grade
○ 11th grade
○ 12th grade, **NO DIPLOMA**
○ **HIGH SCHOOL GRADUATE** - high school
   DIPLOMA or the equivalent (For example: GED)
○ Some college but no degree
○ Associate degree in college - Occupational program
○ Associate degree in college - Academic program
○ Bachelor's degree (For example: BA, AB, BS)
○ Master's degree (For example: MA, MS, MEng,
   MEd, MSW, MBA)   ■
○ Professional school degree
   (For example: MD, DDS, DVM, LLB, JD)
○ Doctorate degree (For example: PhD, EdD)

13. What is . . .'s ancestry or ethnic origin? Ancestry means ethnic origin or descent, "roots", or heritage.
For example: German, Italian, Afro-Amer., Croatian, Cape Verdean, Dominican, Ecuadoran, Haitian, Cajun, French Canadian, Jamaican, Korean, Lebanese, Mexican, Nigerian, Irish, Polish, Slovak, Taiwanese, Thai, Ukrainian, etc.

14a. *If the person was born after April 1, 1985, fill that circle without asking 14a, and go to the next person.*
Did . . . live in this house or apartment 5 years ago (on April 1, 1985)?

○ Born after April 1, 1985 — *Go to questions for the next person*
○ Yes — *Skip to 15a*
○ No

b. Where did . . . live 5 years ago?
(1) Name of U.S. State or foreign country

If outside U.S., print answer above and skip to 15a.
(2) Name of county in the U.S.

(3) Name of city or town in the U.S.

(4) Did . . . live inside the city or town limits?
○ Yes
○ No, lived outside the city/town limits

15a. Does . . . speak a language other than English at home?
○ Yes   ○ No — *Skip to 16*

b. What is this language?

For example: Chinese, Italian, Spanish, Vietnamese

c. How well does . . . speak English — very well, well, not well, or not at all?

○ Very well   ○ Not well
○ Well   ○ Not at all

16. INTERVIEWER CHECK ITEM — *Fill based on question 5.*

○ Born before April 1, 1975 — *Go to 17a*
○ Born April 1, 1975 or later — *Go to questions for the next person*

17a. Has . . . ever been on active-duty military service in the Armed Forces of the United States or ever been in the United States military Reserves or the National Guard? "Active duty" does NOT include training for the military Reserves or National Guard.

○ Yes, now on active duty
○ Yes, on active duty in past, but not now
○ Yes, service in Reserves or National
   Guard only — *Skip to 18*
○ No — *Skip to 18*

b. Did . . . serve on active duty during —*Read each category and fill each circle for which the answer is "Yes."*

○ **September 1980 or later**
○ **May 1975 to August 1980**
○ **Vietnam era (August 1964—April 1975)**
○ **February 1955—July 1964**
○ **Korean conflict (June 1950—January 1955)**
○ **World War II (September 1940—July 1947)**
○ **World War I (April 1917—November 1918)**
○ **Any other time**

c. In total, how many years of active-duty military service has . . . had?
_____ Years

18. Does . . . have a physical, mental, or other health condition that has lasted for 6 or more months and which —
a. Limits the kind or amount of work . . . can do at a job?
○ Yes   ○ No

b. Prevents . . . from working at a job?
○ Yes   ○ No

19. Because of a health condition that has lasted for 6 or more months, does . . . have any difficulty —
a. Going outside the home alone, for example, to shop or visit a doctor's office?
■ Yes   ○ No

b. Taking care of his or her own personal needs, such as bathing, dressing, or getting around inside the home?
○ Yes   ○ No

20. *If this person is a female, ask —*
How many babies has . . . ever had, not counting stillbirths? Do not count stepchildren or children . . . has adopted.
None 1 2 3 4 5 6 7 8 9 10 11 12 or more
○   ○ ○ ○ ○ ○ ○ ○ ○ ○ ○ ○ ○

21a. Did . . . work at any time LAST WEEK, either full time or part time? Work includes part-time work such as delivering papers, or helping without pay in a family business or farm; it also includes active duty in the Armed Forces. Work does NOT include own housework, school work, or volunteer work.

■ Yes   ○ No — *Skip to 25*

b. How many hours did . . . work LAST WEEK at all jobs? Subtract any time off and add any overtime or extra hours worked.
_____ Hours

22. Where did . . . usually work LAST WEEK?
If . . . worked at more than one location, ask —
Where did . . . work most last week?
a. What is the street address?

If the exact address is not known, ask for a description of the location such as the building name or the nearest street or intersection. Do not accept a post office box number.

b. What city, town, or post office is that?

c. Is the work location inside the limits of that city or town?
○ Yes   ○ No, outside the city/town limits

d. What county?

e. In what State?   **f. What ZIP Code?**

23a. What type of transportation did . . . usually use to get to work LAST WEEK? *If more than one method of transportation usually was used during the trip, fill the circle of the one used for most of the distance.*

- ○ Car, truck, or van
- ○ Bus or trolley bus
- ○ Streetcar or trolley car
- ○ Subway or elevated
- ○ Railroad
- ○ Ferryboat
- ○ Taxicab
- ○ Motorcycle
- ○ Bicycle
- ○ Walked
- ○ Worked at home → *Skip to 28*
- ○ Other method

Ask only if "car, truck, or van" is marked in 23a.

b. How many people, including . . . , usually rode to work together LAST WEEK?

- ○ Drove alone
- ○ 2 people
- ○ 3 people
- ○ 4 people
- ○ 5 people
- ○ 6 people
- ○ 7 to 9 people
- ○ 10 or more people

24a. What time did . . . usually leave home to go to work LAST WEEK? "Usually" means on most days last week.

○ a.m. ○ p.m.

b. How many minutes did it usually take . . . to get from home to work LAST WEEK?

Minutes — *Skip to 28*

25. Was . . . on layoff from a job or business LAST WEEK?
If "No," ask — Was . . . temporarily absent or on vacation from a job or business last week?

- ○ Yes, on layoff
- ○ Yes, on vacation, temporary illness, labor dispute, etc.
- ○ No

26a. Has . . . been looking for work during the last 4 weeks?

- ○ Yes
- ○ No — *Skip to 27*

b. Could . . . have taken a job LAST WEEK if one had been offered?
If "No," ask — For what reason?

- ○ No, already has a job
- ○ No, temporarily ill
- ○ No, other reasons (in school, etc.)
- ○ Yes, could have taken a job

27. When did . . . last work, even for a few days?

- ○ 1990
- ○ 1989
- ○ 1988
- ○ 1985 to 1987
- ○ 1980 to 1984 } *Go to 28*
- ○ 1979 or earlier } *Skip to 32*
- ○ Never worked }

28.-30. The following questions ask about the job worked last week. If . . . had more than one job, describe the one . . . worked the most hours. If . . . didn't work, the questions refer to the most recent job or business since 1985.

28a. For whom did . . . work?
If now on active duty in the Armed Forces, fill this circle ──── ○ *and print the branch of the Armed Forces.*
If not Armed Forces, print the name of the company, business or other employer.

b. What kind of business or industry was this? Describe the activity at location where employed.

For example: hospital, newspaper publishing, mail order house, auto engine manufacturing, retail bakery.

c. Is this mainly manufacturing, wholesale trade, retail trade, or something else?

- ○ Manufacturing
- ○ Wholesale trade
- ○ Retail trade
- ○ Other (agriculture, construction, service, government, etc.)

29a. What kind of work was . . . doing?

For example: registered nurse, personnel manager, supervisor of order department, gasoline engine assembler, cake icer.

b. What were . . .'s most important activities or duties?

For example: patient care, directing hiring policies, supervising order clerks, assembling engines, icing cakes.

30. Was . . . — *Read list. Fill ONE circle.*

- ○ Employee of a PRIVATE FOR PROFIT company or business or of an individual, for wages, salary, or commissions
- ○ Employee of a PRIVATE NOT-FOR-PROFIT, tax-exempt, or charitable organization
- ○ Local GOVERNMENT employee (city, county, etc.)
- ○ State GOVERNMENT employee
- ○ Federal GOVERNMENT employee
- ○ SELF-EMPLOYED in own NOT INCORPORATED business, professional practice, or farm
- ○ SELF-EMPLOYED in own INCORPORATED business, professional practice, or farm
- ○ Working WITHOUT PAY in family business or farm

31a. Last year (1989), did . . . work, even for a few days, at a paid job or in a business or farm?

- ○ Yes
- ○ No — *Skip to 32*

b. How many weeks did . . . work in 1989? Count paid vacation, paid sick leave, and military service.

Weeks

c. During the weeks WORKED in 1989, how many hours did . . . usually work each week?

Hours

32. The following questions are about income received during 1989.
If an exact amount is not known, accept a best estimate. If net income in b, c, d or question 33 was a loss, write "Loss" above the dollar amount.

a. Did . . . earn income from wages, salary, commissions, bonuses, or tips? Report the amount before deductions for taxes, bonds, dues, or other items.

- ○ Yes — How much from all jobs? ──→ $ .00
- ○ No
Annual amount — Dollars

b. Did . . . earn any income from (his/her) own nonfarm business, proprietorship, or partnership? Report net income after business expenses.

- ○ Yes — How much? → $ .00
- ○ No
Annual amount — Dollars

c. Did . . . earn any income from (his/her) own farm business? Include earnings as a tenant farmer or sharecropper. Report net income after operating expenses.

- ○ Yes — How much? → $ .00
- ○ No
Annual amount — Dollars

d. Did . . . receive any interest, dividends, net rental or royalty income, or income from estates and trusts? Include even small amounts credited to an account.

- ○ Yes — How much? → $ .00
- ○ No
Annual amount — Dollars

e. Did . . . receive any Social Security or Railroad Retirement payments? Include payments as a retired worker, dependent, or disabled worker.

- ○ Yes — How much? → $ .00
- ○ No
Annual amount — Dollars

f. Did . . . receive any income from government programs for Supplemental Security Income (SSI), Aid to Families with Dependent Children (AFDC), or other public assistance or public welfare payments?

- ○ Yes — How much? → $ .00
- ○ No
Annual amount — Dollars

g. Did . . . receive any income from retirement, survivor, or disability pensions? Include payments from companies, unions, Federal, State, and local governments, and the U.S. military. Do NOT include Social Security.

- ○ Yes — How much? → $ .00
- ○ No
Annual amount — Dollars

h. Did . . . receive any income from Veterans' (VA) payments, unemployment compensation, child support, alimony, or any other regular source of income? Do NOT include lump-sum payments such as money from an inheritance or the sale of a home.

- ○ Yes — How much? → $ .00
- ○ No
Annual amount — Dollars

33. *Do not ask this question if 32a through 32h are complete. Instead, sum these entries and enter the amount below.*
What was . . .'s total income in 1989?

- ○ None   OR $ .00
Annual amount — Dollars

Please turn to the next page and ask the questions for Person 2 on page 2. If this is the last person listed in question 1a on page 1, go to the back of the form.

Appendix B
Populations

Table B.1. United States Standard Population, 1990 Census: Enumerated Population, Standard Million, and Percentage of Population, by Age Group

Age Group	Enumerated Population	Standard Million	% of Population°
Under 1	3,217,312	12,938	1.29
1 and 2	7,764,147	31,222	3.12
3 and 4	7,372,984	29,649	2.96
5	3,689,533	14,837	1.48
6	3,577,632	14,387	1.44
7–9	10,832,014	43,559	4.36
10 and 11	7,108,692	28,586	2.86
12 and 13	6,762,150	27,193	2.72
14	3,243,107	13,042	1.30
15	3,321,609	13,357	1.34
16	3,301,890	13,278	1.33
17	3,410,062	13,713	1.37
18	3,611,238	14,522	1.45
19	4,076,216	16,392	1.64
20	4,009,414	16,123	1.61
21	3,817,220	15,350	1.54
22–24	11,193,678	45,014	4.50
25–29	21,313,045	85,707	8.57
30–34	21,862,887	87,918	8.79
35–39	19,963,117	80,278	8.03
40–44	17,615,786	70,839	7.08
45–49	13,872,573	55,786	5.58
50–54	11,350,513	45,644	4.56
55–59	10,531,766	42,352	4.24
60–61	4,228,303	17,003	1.70
62–64	6,387,861	25,688	2.57

Table B.1. (continued)

Age Group	Enumerated Population	Standard Million	% of Population°
65–69	10,111,735	40,663	4.07
70–74	7,991,823	32,138	3.21
75–79	6,121,369	24,616	2.46
80–84	3,933,739	15,819	1.58
85+	3,080,165	12,387	1.24
Total	248,673,580	1,000,000	100.00

° Percentage may not equal 100% due to rounding up of numbers.

Table B.2. United States Population, 1990 Census: Enumerated Population, Standard Million, and Percentage of Population, by Selected Age Groups

Age Group	Enumerated Population	Standard Million	% of Population
0–4	18,354,443	73,809	7.38
5–9	18,099,179	72,783	7.28
10–14	17,113,949	68,821	6.88
15–19	17,721,015	71,262	7.13
20–24	19,020,312	76,487	7.65
25–29	21,313,045	85,707	8.57
30–34	21,862,887	87,918	8.79
35–44	37,578,903	151,117	15.11
45–54	25,223,086	101,430	10.14
55–64	21,147,930	85,043	8.51
65+	31,238,831	125,623	12.56
Total	248,673,580	1,000,000	100.00

Table B.3. United States Standard Population, 1990 Census, by Age, Sex, and Race/Ethnicity

Age Group	White Males	White Females	Black Males	Black Females	Asian Males	Asian Females	Other Males	Other Females
Under 1	1,232,872	1,171,386	242,400	237,622	47,604	45,856	103,622	99,861
1 and 2	2,945,331	2,793,998	607,662	593,399	131,890	124,821	246,344	235,468
3 and 4	2,826,278	2,679,625	558,433	546,386	121,852	117,822	225,493	216,468
5	1,421,766	1,346,446	275,929	269,626	61,701	60,087	109,145	104,176
6	1,383,042	1,312,121	263,945	258,345	60,486	58,977	102,374	98,888
7–9	4,185,723	3,967,170	810,391	792,873	179,646	175,236	307,191	294,449
10 and 11	2,745,346	2,591,137	550,409	538,037	115,416	110,990	194,712	184,840
12 and 13	2,610,071	2,473,496	516,846	507,846	110,299	106,903	184,168	178,354
14	1,251,309	1,182,199	247,153	241,299	55,410	52,534	90,281	87,194
15	1,283,835	1,210,057	253,591	245,923	58,385	54,278	91,621	88,179
16	1,271,496	1,198,352	256,012	247,997	59,630	55,847	92,537	87,133
17	1,313,056	1,232,117	266,726	255,565	60,945	56,772	99,029	89,907
18	1,395,825	1,335,222	274,060	271,925	64,788	60,522	109,086	94,012
19	1,581,359	1,521,384	291,874	294,820	68,669	63,925	117,116	99,922
20	1,557,979	1,502,020	273,585	279,680	70,127	64,567	124,232	102,100
21	1,487,818	1,433,616	253,358	259,894	67,260	61,919	121,953	98,001
22–24	4,342,583	4,199,896	731,683	780,753	188,595	179,790	371,380	301,974
25–29	8,384,815	8,253,729	1,285,760	1,422,005	342,628	348,441	595,259	504,831
30–34	8,699,545	8,651,968	1,250,610	1,431,114	349,807	376,376	494,227	438,572
35–39	8,054,129	8,024,477	1,083,051	1,253,715	316,522	353,296	375,947	348,798
40–44	7,227,231	7,279,159	865,660	1,010,402	266,792	305,402	271,107	263,879
45–49	5,736,583	5,849,129	642,441	763,325	195,406	210,184	189,174	189,523
50–54	4,657,384	4,847,487	531,976	647,035	152,085	159,566	136,405	141,861
55–59	4,330,811	4,637,605	456,919	575,830	113,509	137,124	103,777	114,362
60–61	1,733,997	1,915,791	169,321	221,011	39,560	52,076	34,954	40,148
62–64	2,600,787	2,960,548	244,924	326,363	54,579	72,302	44,733	53,684
65–69	4,013,229	4,886,408	362,942	500,103	79,518	98,979	57,320	70,526
70–74	3,055,729	4,070,835	254,699	385,716	54,300	67,934	32,078	44,262
75–79	2,154,399	3,330,626	178,540	302,730	36,801	43,338	21,568	32,215
80–84	1,227,102	2,325,593	100,659	192,979	21,429	22,421	12,347	19,093
85+	764,450	2,023,602	68,592	161,591	12,399	17,339	8,983	14,004
Total	97,475,880	102,207,199	14,170,151	15,815,909	3,558,038	3,715,624	5,068,163	4,736,684

**Table B.4. United States Standard Population, 1990 Census,
by Households and Race/Ethnicity**

Households by Type

Total households		91,947,410
Family households (families)		64,517,947
Married-couple families		50,708,322
Total households (percent)	55.10	
Other family, male householder		3,143,582
Other family, female householder		10,666,043
Nonfamily households		27,429,463
Total households (percent)	29.80	
Householder living alone		22,580,420
Householder 65 years and over		8,824,845
Persons living in households		242,012,129
Persons per household		2.63

Group Quarters

Persons living in group quarters	6,697,744
Institutionalized persons	3,334,018
Others persons in group quarters	3,363,726

Race and Hispanic Origin

White		199,686,070
Black		29,986,060
Total population (percent)	12.10	
American Indian, Eskimo, or Aleut		1,959,234
Total population (percent)	0.80	
Asian or Pacific Islander		7,273,662
Total population (percent)	2.90	
Other race		9,804,847
Hispanic origin (of any race)		22,354,059
Total population (percent)	9.00	
Total housing units		102,263,678

Occupancy and Tenure

Occupied housing units		91,947,410
Owner occupied		59,024,811
Owner occupied (percent)	64.20	
Renter occupied		32,922,599
Vacant housing units		10,316,268
For seasonal or occasional use		3,081,923
Homeowner vacancy rate (percent)	2.10	
Rental vacancy rate (percent)	8.50	
Persons per owner-occupied unit		2.75
Persons per renter-occupied unit		2.42

Table B.4. (continued)

Units with over one person per room	4,548,799
Units in Structure	
One unit, detached	60,383,409
One unit, attached	5,378,243
Two to four units	9,876,408
Five to nine units	4,935,841
Ten or more units	13,168,769
Mobile home, trailer, or other	8,521,009
Value	
Specified owner-occupied units	44,918,000
Less than $50,000	11,402,522
$50,000 to $99,000	16,957,458
$100,000 to $149,000	6,773,257
$150,000 to $199,000	4,017,162
$200,000 to $299,999	3,376,901
$300,000 or more	2,390,700
Median (dollars)	79,100
Contract Rent	
Specified renter-occupied units paying cash rent	30,490,535
Less than $250	7,478,207
$250 to $499	14,371,897
$500 to $749	6,188,367
$750 to $999	1,626,608
$1,000 or more	825,456
Median (dollars)	374

Race and Hispanic Origin of Householder		
Occupied housing units		91,947,410
White		76,880,105
Black		9,976,161
Occupied units (percent)	10.80	
American Indian, Eskimo, or Aleut		591,372
Occupied units (percent)	0.60	
Asian or Pacific Islander		2,013,735
Occupied units (percent)	2.20	
Other race		2,486,037
Hispanic origin (of any race)		6,001,718
Occupied units (percent)	6.50	

Appendix C
Additional Practice Problems

Practice Problem One

Figure the missing rates for the following table (round decimals to hundredths).

Table C.1. Ohio Vital Statistics, 1988

Vital Event	Number			Rate		
	Total	White	Black	Total	White	Black
Live births	160,344	132,988	25,511	(a)	(q)	(ee)
Low births	10,995	7,566	3,319	(b)	(r)	(ff)
Illegitimate births	42,372	23,920	18,224	(c)	(s)	(gg)
Deaths (total)	100,325	89,604	10,549	(d)	(t)	(hh)
Select causes						
Heart disease	37,776	34,319	3,399	(e)	(u)	(ii)
Cancer	23,375	20,780	2,558	(f)	(v)	(jj)
Stroke	7,122	6,403	708	(g)	(w)	(kk)
COPD	4,259	3,957	296	(h)	(x)	(ll)
Accidents	3,785	3,293	478	(i)	(y)	(mm)
Infant deaths	1,555	1,144	403	(j)	(z)	(nn)
Neonatal deaths	978	730	242	(k)	(aa)	(oo)
Fetal deaths	1,162	894	257	(l)	(bb)	(pp)
Perinatal deaths	2,140	1,624	499	(m)	(cc)	(qq)
Maternal deaths	5	2	3	(n)	(dd)	(rr)
Marriages	97,881	0	0	(o)		
Divorces	49,244	0	0	(p)		

Table C.1. (continued)

Population:		Live birthrates per 1,000 population
Total	10,797,630	Low births and illegitimate birthrates per 1,000 live births
White	9,597,458	Death, all causes, and selected causes rates per 100,000 population
Black	1,076,748	Infant, neonatal, and fetal death rates per 1,000 live births
Other	123,424	Perinatal death rates determined by perinatal deaths divided by fetal deaths and total births × 1,000
		Maternal death rate per 10,000 live births
		Marriages and divorces rates per 1,000 population

Source: Ohio Vital Statistics, 1989, Ohio Department of Health

Table C.1A. Ohio Vital Statistics, 1988—Answers

Vital Event	Number			Rate		
	Total	White	Black	Total	White	Black
Live births	160,344	132,988	25,511	14.85	13.86	23.69
Low births	10,995	7,566	3,319	68.57	56.89	130.10
Illegitimate births	42,372	23,920	18,224	264.26	179.87	714.36
Deaths (total)	100,325	89,604	10,549	929.14	933.62	979.71
Select causes						
Heart disease	37,776	34,319	3,399	349.85	357.58	315.67
Cancer	23,375	20,780	2,558	216.48	216.52	237.57
Stroke	7,122	6,403	708	65.96	66.72	65.75
COPD	4,259	3,957	296	39.44	41.23	27.49
Accidents	3,785	3,293	478	35.05	34.31	44.39
Infant deaths	1,555	1,144	403	9.70	8.60	15.80
Neonatal deaths	978	730	242	6.10	5.49	9.49
Fetal deaths	1,162	894	257	7.25	6.72	10.07
Perinatal deaths	2,140	1,624	499	13.25	12.13	19.37
Maternal deaths	5	2	3	0.31	0.15	1.18
Marriages	97,881	0	0	9.07	0.00	0.00
Divorces	49,244	0	0	4.56	0.00	0.00

Rationale for Ohio Vital Statistics Rates in Table C.1

Item (a) is determined by dividing total live births by total population times 1,000 (base).
Item (q) is determined by dividing white live births by white population times 1,000.
Item (ee) is determined by dividing black live births by black population times 1,000.

Item (b) is determined by dividing total low births by total live births times 1,000.

Item (r) is determined by dividing white low births by white live births times 1,000.
Item (ff) is determined by dividing black low births by black live births times 1,000.

Item (c) is determined by dividing total illegitimate births by total live births times 1,000.
Item (s) is determined by dividing white illegitimate births by white live births times 1,000.
Item (gg) is determined by dividing black illegitimate births by black live births times 1,000.

Item (d) is determined by dividing total deaths by total population times 100,000 (base).
Item (t) is determined by dividing white deaths by white population times 100,000.
Item (hh) is determined by dividing black deaths by black population times 100,000.

Items (e–i) are determined by dividing select total cause by total population times 100,000.
Items (u–y) are determined by dividing select white cause by white population times 100,000.
Items (ii–mm) are determined by dividing select black cause by black population times 100,000.

Items (j and k) are determined by dividing total deaths by total live births times 1,000 (base).
Items (z and aa) are determined by dividing white deaths by white live births times 1,000.
Items (nn and oo) are determined by dividing black deaths by black live births times 1,000.

Item (l) is determined by dividing total fetal deaths by total live births times 1,000 (base).
Item (bb) is determined by dividing white fetal deaths by white live births times 1,000.
Item (pp) is determined by dividing black fetal deaths by black live births times 1,000.

Item (m) is determined by the number of perinatal deaths divided by fetal deaths and total live births times 1,000 (base).
Item (cc) is determined by the number of white perinatal deaths divided by white fetal deaths and total live births times 1,000.
Item (qq) is determined by the number of black perinatal deaths divided by black fetal deaths and black births times 1,000.

Item (n) is determined by dividing total maternal deaths by total live births times 10,000 (base).
Item (dd) is determined by dividing white maternal deaths by white live births times 10,000.
Item (rr) is determined by dividing black maternal deaths by black live births times 10,000.

Items (o) and (p) are determined by dividing the total number by the total population times 1,000 (base).

Practice Problem Two

Figure the missing rates for the following table (round decimals to hundredths).

Table C.2. Missouri Vital Statistics, 1988

Vital Event	Number			Rate		
	Total	White	Nonwhite	Total	White	Nonwhite
Live births	76,101	62,397	13,704	(a)	(q)	(dd)
Low births	5,251	3,494	1,757	(b)	(r)	(ee)
Illegitimate births	19,057	9,878	9,179	(c)	(s)	(ff)
Deaths (total)	50,619	45,384	5,235	(d)	(t)	(gg)
Select causes						
Heart disease	18,433	16,845	1,588	(e)	(u)	(hh)
Cancer	10,913	9,750	1,163	(f)	(v)	(ii)
Stroke	3,607	3,271	336	(g)	(w)	(jj)
COPD	2,096	1,980	116	(h)	(x)	(kk)
Accidents	2,127	1,890	237	(i)	(y)	(ll)
Infant deaths	770	562	208	(j)	(z)	(mm)
Neonatal deaths	486	351	135	(k)	(aa)	(nn)
Fetal deaths	513	0	0	(l)		
Perinatal deaths	999	0	0	(m)		
Maternal deaths	5	0	0	(n)		
Marriages	50,330	44,767	5,563	(o)	(bb)	(oo)
Divorces	24,948	22,123	2,825	(p)	(cc)	(pp)

Population:

White   4,529,221

Nonwhite   611,779

Total   5,141,000

Live birthrates per 1,000 population

Low birth and illegitimate birthrates per 1,000 live births

Death, all causes, and selected causes rates per 100,000 population

Infant, neonatal, and fetal death rates per 1,000 live births

Perinatal death rates determined by perinatal deaths divided by fetal deaths and total births × 1,000

Maternal death rate per 10,000 live births

Marriages and divorces rates per 1,000 population

Source: Missouri Vital Statistics, 1989, Missouri Department of Health

Table C.2A. Missouri Vital Statistics, 1988—Answers

Vital Event	Number			Rate		
	Total	White	Nonwhite	Total	White	Nonwhite
Live births	76,101	62,397	13,704	14.80	13.78	22.40
Low births	5,251	3,494	1,757	69.00	56.00	128.21
Illegitimate births	19,057	9,878	9,179	250.42	158.31	669.80

Table C.2A. (continued)

Vital Event	Number			Rate		
	Total	White	Nonwhite	Total	White	Nonwhite
Deaths (total)	50,619	45,384	5,235	984.61	1,002.03	855.70
Select causes						
Heart disease	18,433	16,845	1,588	358.55	371.92	259.57
Cancer	10,913	9,750	1,163	212.27	215.27	190.10
Stroke	3,607	3,271	336	70.16	72.22	54.92
COPD	2,096	1,980	116	40.77	43.72	18.96
Accidents	2,127	1,890	237	41.37	41.73	38.74
Infant deaths	770	562	208	10.12	9.01	15.18
Neonatal deaths	486	351	135	6.39	5.63	9.85
Fetal deaths	513	0	0	6.74	0.00	0.00
Perinatal deaths	999	0	0	13.04	0.00	0.00
Maternal deaths	5	0	0	0.66	0.00	0.00
Marriages	50,330	44,767	5,563	9.79	9.88	9.09
Divorces	24,948	22,123	2,825	4.85	4.88	4.62

Rationale for Missouri Vital Statistics Rates in Table C.2

Item (a) is determined by dividing total live births by total population times 1,000 (base).
Item (q) is determined by dividing white live births by white population times 1,000.
Item (dd) is determined by dividing nonwhite live births by nonwhite population times 1,000.

Item (b) is determined by dividing total low births by total live births times 1,000.
Item (r) is determined by dividing white low births by white live births times 1,000.
Item (ee) is determined by dividing nonwhite low births by nonwhite live births times 1,000.

Item (c) is determined by dividing total illegitimate births by total live births times 1,000.
Item (s) is determined by dividing white illegitimate births by white live births times 1,000.
Item (ff) is determined by dividing nonwhite illegitimate births by nonwhite live births times 1,000.

Item (d) is determined by dividing total deaths by total population times 100,000 (base).
Item (t) is determined by dividing white deaths by white population times 100,000.
Item (gg) is determined by dividing nonwhite deaths by nonwhite population times 100,000.

Items (e–i) are determined by dividing select total cause by total population times 100,000.

Items (u–y) are determined by dividing select white cause by white population times 100,000.

Items (hh–ll) are determined by dividing select nonwhite cause by nonwhite population times 100,000.

Items (j and k) are determined by dividing total deaths by total live births times 1,000 (base).

Items (z and aa) are determined by dividing white deaths by white live births times 1,000.

Items (mm and nn) are determined by dividing nonwhite deaths by nonwhite live births times 1,000.

Item (l) is determined by dividing total fetal deaths by total live births times 1,000.

Item (m) is determined by the number of perinatal deaths divided by fetal deaths and total live births times 1,000.

Item (n) is determined by dividing total maternal deaths by total live births times 10,000 (base).

Items (o) and (p) are determined by dividing the total number by the total population times 1,000 (base).

Items (bb) and (cc) are determined by dividing the white numbers by the white population times 1,000.

Items (oo) and (pp) are determined by dividing the nonwhite numbers by the nonwhite population times 1,000.

Practice Problem Three

Figure the deaths per one hundred thousand for the following table.

Table C.3. Population Distribution and Age-Specific Death Rates for Alaska and Florida, 1987°

Age Group	Alaska			Florida		
	Deaths	Population	Deaths/ 100,000 (ASDR)	Deaths	Population	Deaths/ 100,000 (ASDR)
0–4	162	40,000	(a)	2,049	546,000	(g)
5–19	107	128,000	(b)	1,195	1,982,000	(h)
20–44	449	172,000	(c)	5,097	2,676,000	(i)
45–64	451	58,000	(d)	19,904	1,807,000	(j)
65+	444	9,000	(e)	63,505	1,444,000	(k)
Total	1,615	407,000	(f)	91,760	8,455,000	(l)

°Data are fictitious.

Table C.3A. Population Distribution and Age-Specific Death Rates for Alaska and Florida, 1987—Answers

Age Group	Alaska			Florida		
	Deaths	Population	Deaths/ 100,000 (ASDR)	Deaths	Population	Deaths/ 100,000 (ASDR)
0–4	162	40,000	405.00	2,049	546,000	375.27
5–19	107	128,000	83.59	1,195	1,982,000	60.29
20–44	449	172,000	261.05	5,097	2,676,000	190.47
45–64	451	58,000	777.59	19,904	1,807,000	1,101.49
65+	444	9,000	4,933.33	63,505	1,444,000	4,397.85
Total	1,615	407,000	396.81	91,760	8,455,000	1,085.27

Rationale for Problems in Table C.3

To figure items (a) through (f), divide the number of deaths in Alaska per age group by the population in that age group times the base (100,000). For example, for item (a), 162/40,000 × 100,000 = 405.

To figure items (g) through (l), divide the number of deaths in Florida per age group by the population in that age group times the base (100,000). For example, for item (g), 2,049/546,000 × 100,000 = 375.30.

Practice Problem Four

Figure the expected deaths for the following table.

Table C.4. Age-Specific Death Rates and Expected Deaths for Alaska and Florida, 1990 (Using the Direct Method and Based on the 1990 U.S. Standard Million)°

Age Group	1990 U.S. Standard Million	Alaska		Florida	
		ASDR	Expected Deaths	ASDR	Expected Deaths
0–4	73,809	405.00	(a)	375.30	(f)
5–19	212,866	83.60	(b)	60.30	(g)
20–34	250,112	261.00	(c)	190.50	(h)
35–64	337,591	777.00	(d)	1,101.50	(i)
65+	125,622	4,933.30	(e)	4,397.90	(j)
Total	1,000,000				

°Data are fictitious.

Table C.4A. Age-Specific Death Rates and Expected Deaths for Alaska and Florida, 1990 (Using the Direct Method and Based on the 1990 U.S. Standard Million)—Answers

Age Group	1990 U.S. Standard Million	Alaska		Florida	
		ASDR	Expected Deaths	ASDR	Expected Deaths
0–4	73,809	405.00	29.89	375.30	27.70
5–19	212,866	83.60	17.80	60.30	12.84
20–34	250,112	261.00	65.28	190.50	47.65
35–64	337,591	777.00	262.31	1,101.50	371.86
65+	125,622	4,933.30	619.73	4,397.90	552.47
Total	1,000,000				

Rationale for Problems in Table C.4

To figure items (a) through (e), multiply the ASDR times the U.S. Standard Million and divide by 1,000,000. For example, for the Alaska age group 0–4, 405.00 × 73,809/ 1,000,000 = 29.89.

To figure items (f) through (j), multiply the ASDR times the U.S. Standard Million and divide by 1,000,000. For example, for the Florida age group 0–4, 375.30 × 73,809/ 1,000,000 = 27.70.

To figure items (k) and (l), add columns.

Practice Problem Five

Figure the expected deaths for the following table.

Table C.5. Age-Specific Death Rates and Expected Deaths for Alaska and Florida, 1990 (Using the Direct Method and Based on the 1990 U.S. Percentage of Population)[*]

Age Group	1990 U.S. Percentage of Population	Alaska		Florida	
		ASDR	Expected Deaths	ASDR	Expected Deaths
0–4	7.38	405.00	(a)	375.30	(f)
5–19	21.41	83.60	(b)	60.30	(g)
20–34	25.01	261.00	(c)	190.50	(h)
35–64	33.75	777.00	(d)	1,101.50	(i)
65+	12.56	4,933.30	(e)	4,397.90	(j)
Total	100.00				

[*]Data are fictitious.

Table C.5A. Age-Specific Death Rates and Expected Deaths for Alaska and Florida, 1990 (Using the Direct Method and Based on the 1990 U.S. Percentage of Population)—Answers

Age Group	1990 U.S. Population Percent	Alaska ASDR	Alaska Expected Deaths	Florida ASDR	Florida Expected Deaths
0–4	7.38	405.00	29.89	375.30	27.70
5–19	21.41	83.60	17.90	60.30	12.91
20–34	25.01	261.00	65.28	190.50	47.64
35–64	33.75	777.00	262.24	1,101.50	371.76
65+	12.56	4,933.30	619.62	4,397.90	552.38
Total	100.00				

Rationale for Problems in Table C.5

To figure items (a) through (e), multiply the ASDR times the U.S. Percentage. For example, for the Alaska 0–4 age group, $405.00 \times 7.38\%$ (or .0738) = 29.89.

To figure items (f) through (j), multiply the ASDR times the U.S. Percentage. For example, for the Florida 0–4 age group, 375.30 times 7.38% (or .0738) = 27.70.

You should note that you may have slightly different answers due to the fact that the percentage you are using for the standard population has been rounded up or down.

Practice Problem Six

Figure the death rate per one thousand for the following table.

Table C.6. Populations, Deaths, and Death Rates for Bonehead Village and Dope City, by Community and Age*

Age Group	Bonehead Village Population	Bonehead Village Deaths	Bonehead Village Death Rate/1,000	Dope City Population	Dope City Deaths	Dope City Death Rate/1,000
Under 1	1,000	15	(a)	5,000	100	(h)
1–14	3,000	3	(b)	20,000	10	(i)
15–34	6,000	6	(c)	35,000	35	(j)
35–54	13,000	52	(d)	17,000	85	(k)
55–64	7,000	105	(e)	8,000	160	(l)
65+	20,000	1,600	(f)	15,000	1,350	(m)
Total	50,000	1,781	(g)	100,000	1,740	(n)

*Data are fictitious.

Table C.6A. Populations, Deaths, and Death Rates for Bonehead Village and Dope City, by Community and Age—Answers

Age Group	Bonehead Village			Dope City		
	Population	Deaths	Death Rate/1,000	Population	Deaths	Death Rate/1,000
Under 1	1,000	15	15.00	5,000	100	20.00
1–14	3,000	3	1.00	20,000	10	0.50
15–34	6,000	6	1.00	35,000	35	1.00
35–54	13,000	52	4.00	17,000	85	5.00
55–64	7,000	105	15.00	8,000	160	20.00
65+	20,000	1,600	80.00	15,000	1,350	90.00
Total	50,000	1,781	35.62	100,000	1,740	17.40

Rationale for Problems in Table C.6

To figure items (a) through (g), divide the age group deaths by the age group population and then multiply times 1,000. For example, for the under 1 age group in Bonehead Village, 15 (deaths)/1,000 (the population of that age group) × 1,000 (the base) = 15.00.

To figure items (h) through (n), multiply the age group deaths by the age group population and multiply times 1,000. For example, for the under 1 age group in Dope City, 100 (deaths)/5,000 (population in age group) × 1,000 = 20.00.

Practice Problem Seven

Figure the expected deaths for the following table.

Table C.7. Age-Specific Death Rates and Expected Deaths for Bonehead Village and Dope City (Using Pooled Population)°

Age Group	Pooled Population	Bonehead Village		Dope City	
		ASDR	Expected Deaths	ASDR	Expected Deaths
Under 1	6,000	15.00	(a)	20.00	(h)
1–14	23,000	1.00	(b)	0.50	(i)
15–34	41,000	1.00	(c)	1.00	(j)
35–54	30,000	4.00	(d)	5.00	(k)
55–64	15,000	15.00	(e)	20.00	(l)
65+	35,000	80.00	(f)	90.00	(m)
Total	150,000	35.60	(g)	17.40	(n)
Age Adjusted		(o)		(p)	

°Data are fictitious.

Table C.7A. Age-Specific Death Rates and Expected Deaths for Bonehead Village and Dope City (Using Pooled Population)—Answers

Age Group	Pooled Population	Bonehead Village ASDR	Bonehead Village Expected Deaths	Dope City ASDR	Dope City Expected Deaths
Under 1	6,000	15.00	0.60	20.00	0.80
1–14	23,000	1.00	0.15	0.50	0.08
15–34	41,000	1.00	0.27	1.00	0.27
35–54	30,000	4.00	0.80	5.00	1.00
55–64	15,000	15.00	1.50	20.00	2.00
65+	35,000	80.00	18.67	90.00	21.00
Total	150,000	35.60	21.99	17.40	25.15
Age Adjusted		0.15		0.17	

Rationale for Problems in Table C.7

To figure items (a) through (f), multiply death rate of Bonehead Village times standard pooled population of age group and divide by the total population (150,000). For example, for (a), 15.00 × 6,000/150,000 = .60.

To figure items (h) through (m), multiply death rate of Dope City times standard pooled population of age group and divide by total population (150,000). For example, for (h), 20.00 × 6,000/150,000 = .80.

To figure item (g), add items (a) through (f).

To figure item (n), add items (h) through (m).

To figure item (o), divide (g) by total population (150,000) and multiply by base (1,000): 21.99/150,000 × 1,000 = .15.

To figure item (p), divide (n) by total population and multiply by base: 25.15/150,000 × 1,000 = .17.

Practice Problem Eight

Part 1

Figure the missing percentages in the following tables. Round off to the nearest ten-thousandth.

Table C.8. Worksheet for Ratio, Proportion, and Percentage

Age Group	Population	Proportion/Percentage of Population
0–4	8,638	
5–14	16,789	

Table C.8. (continued)

Age Group	Population	Proportion/Percentage of Population
15–24	22,214	
25–34	16,543	
35–44	12,654	
45–54	9,888	
55–64	8,564	
65+	4,075	
Total	99,365	

Age Group	No. of Cases	Proportion/Percentage of Disease
0–4	22	
5–14	39	
15–24	111	
25–34	93	
35–44	76	
45–54	22	
55–64	65	
65+	12	
Total	440	

Part 2

Use the information from the following table to answer the questions below. This is a breakdown of students who are suffering from studyitis at Pinhead University.

Dormitory	Sex	Populations of Dorms	No. of Cases
1	F	80	19
2	F	112	2
3	F	89	0
4	F	111	1
5	F	53	5
6	M	35	0
7	M	63	0
8	F	103	4

9	M	35	1
10	M	37	0
11	F	34	1
12	M	62	13
13	M	32	1
14	M	10	0
Total		856	47

1. What is the ratio of males to females in these dormitories?
2. What is the ratio of males to females who have fallen ill?
3. What is the ratio of ill students to well students?
4. What is the ratio of ill females to well females?
5. What is the ratio of ill males to well males?

Part 3

Use the following information to answer the questions below.

Total midyear population	80,000
Population 45 years of age and over	20,000
Number of infants born alive	2,000
Fetal deaths (reported)	32
Maternal deaths	1
Total deaths	648
Deaths under 1 year of age	42
Deaths of persons 45 and over	300
From heart disease	98
From cancer	60
From stroke	48
From all other causes	94

1. Using the number of deaths of people 45 years and over, what is the proportion/percentage of deaths from cancer of those individuals?
2. Using the number of deaths of people 45 years and over, what is the proportion/percentage of deaths from stroke of those individuals?
3. What is the ratio of deaths from heart disease to deaths from cancer for those 45 years and over?
4. What is the ratio of deaths from heart disease to deaths from all other causes for those 45 years and over?
5. What is the ratio of deaths from cancer to deaths from strokes for those 45 years and over?
6. What is the ratio of deaths of those 45 years of age and older to the deaths of those under 45 years of age?

Part 1. Answers

Table C.8A. Worksheet for Ratio, Proportion, and Percentage—Answers

Age Group	Population	Proportion/Percentage of Population (Rationale and Answer)
0–4	8,638	8,638/99,365 = .0869 (8.7%)
5–14	16,789	16,789/99,365 = .16896 (16.9%)
15–24	22,214	22,214/99,365 = .22355 (22.4%)
25–34	16,543	16,543/99,365 = .16649 (16.6%)
35–44	12,654	12,654/99,365 = .12734 (12.7%)
45–54	9,888	9,888/99,365 = .0995 (10.0%)
55–64	8,564	8,564/99,365 = .0862 (8.6%)
65+	4,075	4,075/99,365 = .0410 (4.1%)
Total	99,365	

Age Group	No. of Cases	Proportion/Percentage of Disease (Rationale and Answer)
0–4	22	22/8,638 = .0026 (.26%)
5–14	39	39/16,789 = .0023 (.23%)
15–24	111	111/22,214 = .0050 (.50%)
25–34	93	93/16,543 = .0060 (.60%)
35–44	76	76/12,654 = .0060 (.60%)
45–54	22	22/9,888 = .0020 (.22%)
55–64	65	64/8,564 = .0078 (.80%)
65+	12	12/4,075 = .0030 (.30%)
Total	440	

Part 2. Answers

1. There are 274 males and 582 females; the ratio is 274/582 = .47 males to 1.00 female. In other words, for ever 1.00 female, there are .47 males.
2. Among the 274 males, 15 males have become ill; of the 582 females, 32 have become ill. The ratio of ill males to ill females is 15/32 = .4688 males to 1.00 female. In other words, for every 1.00 female that has become ill, .4688 males have become ill.
3. Among the 856 students, 47 have become ill. The ratio of ill to well students would

be 47/856 = .0549 to 1.00. In other words, for every 1.00 student, .0549 have become ill.

4. Of the 582 females, 32 have become ill. The ratio of ill females to well females would be 32/582 = .0549 to 1.00. In other words, for every 1.00 well female, .0549 have become ill.

5. Of the 274 males, 15 have become ill. The ratio of ill males to well males would be 15/274 = .0547 to 1.00. In other words, for every 1.00 well male, .0547 have fallen ill.

Part 3. Answers

1. There were 300 deaths of people 45 and over; 60 of those deaths were from cancer. To figure the proportion of deaths, the formula is 60/300 = .20 (20%).

2. Of the 300 deaths, 48 were from strokes. The formula is 48/300 = .16 (16%).

3. There were 98 people over 45 who died from heart disease and 60 who died from cancer. The ratio of heart disease to cancer would be 98/60 = 1.63. In other words, for every 1.00 death from cancer, 1.63 died from heart disease.

4. Ninety-eight people died from heart disease and 94 died from all other causes. The ratio is 98/94 = 1.04 to 1.00. In other words, for every person that died from all other causes, 1.04 died from heart disease.

5. Sixty people died from cancer and 48 died from stroke. The ratio is 60/48 = 1.25 to 1.00. In other words, for every 1.00 person over 45 who died from stroke, 1.25 died from cancer.

6. Three hundred people 45 and over died and 348 under 45 died (for the total deaths of 648). The ratio of deaths of those 45 and older to those under 45 would be 300/348 = .86 to 1.00. In other words, for every 1.00 person under 45 that died, .86 over 45 died.

Practice Problem Nine

Figure the missing rates in tables C.9, C.10, and C.11 using the following total populations of counties, cities, and balances of counties in Ohio.

Ohio	10,797,630
Columbia County	113,572
E. Liverpool	16,687
E. Palestine	5,306
Salem	12,839
Wellville	5,095
Balance	73,615
Mahoning County	289,487
Campbell	11,619
Canfield	5,535
Sebring	5,078
Struthers	13,624
Youngstown	115,427

Balance	138,204
Trumbull County	241,863
Cortland	5,011
Girard	12,517
Hubbard	9,245
Newton Falls	4,960
Niles	23,089
Warren	56,629
Youngstown	9
Balance	130,404

Table C.9. Live Births Classified by Race, Number, and Rate, by County, City, and Balance of County, Ohio, 1985

County, City, and Balance of County	Live Births	Number White	Black	Rate°
Ohio	160,433	135,666	24,767	(a)
Columbia County	1,546	1,522	24	(b)
E. Liverpool	249	238	11	(c)
E. Palestine	75	75	0	14.10
Salem	196	194	2	15.20
Wellville	69	65	4	13.50
Balance	957	950	7	(d)
Mahoning County	3,679	2,809	870	(e)
Campbell	124	100	24	(f)
Canfield	81	81	0	14.60
Sebring	72	72	0	14.20
Struthers	144	137	7	10.60
Youngstown	1,612	812	800	(g)
Balance	1,626	1,587	39	(h)
Trumbull County	3,249	2,907	342	(i)
Cortland	124	123	1	(j)
Girard	191	183	8	15.30
Hubbard	111	110	1	12.00
Newton Falls	89	89	0	(k)
Niles	312	302	10	13.50
Warren	1,038	756	282	(l)
Youngstown	1	1	0	0.00
Balance	1,383	1,343	40	(m)

°Per 1,000 population of particular community

Table C.9A. Live Births Classified by Race, Number, and Rate, by County, City, and Balance of County, Ohio, 1985—Answers

County, City, and Balance of County	Live Births	Number White	Black	Rate
Ohio	160,433	135,666	24,767	14.86
Columbia County	1,546	1,522	24	13.61
E. Liverpool	249	238	11	14.92
E. Palestine	75	75	0	14.13
Salem	196	194	2	15.27
Wellville	69	65	4	13.54
Balance	957	950	7	13.00
Mahoning County	3,679	2,809	870	12.71
Campbell	124	100	24	10.67
Canfield	81	81	0	14.63
Sebring	72	72	0	14.18
Struthers	144	137	7	10.57
Youngstown	1,612	812	800	13.97
Balance	1,626	1,587	39	11.77
Trumbull County	3,249	2,907	342	13.43
Cortland	124	123	1	24.75
Girard	191	183	8	15.26
Hubbard	111	110	1	12.01
Newton Falls	89	89	0	17.94
Niles	312	302	10	13.51
Warren	1,038	756	282	18.33
Youngstown	1	1	0	111.11
Balance	1,383	1,343	40	10.61

Table C.10. Premature Births Classified by Race, Number, and Rate, by County, City, and Balance of County, Ohio, 1985

County, City, and Balance of County	Premature Births	Number White	Black	Rate° Total	White	Black
Ohio	10,700	7,837	2,874	(n)	(o)	116.00
Columbia County	87	86	1	56.30	56.50	(p)
E. Liverpool	17	17	0	68.30	71.40	0.00
E. Palestine	5	5	0	66.70	66.70	0.00
Salem	10	10	0	51.00	51.50	0.00

Table C.10. (continued)

Wellville	11	10	1	159.40	153.80	250.00
Balance	44	44	0	46.00	46.30	0.00
Mahoning County	290	153	137	(q)	54.50	(r)
Campbell	6	3	3	48.40	30.00	125.00
Canfield	6	6	0	74.10	74.10	0.00
Sebring	0	0	0	0.00	0.00	0.00
Struthers	6	5	1	41.70	36.50	(s)
Youngstown	182	56	126	(t)	67.30	(u)
Balance	90	83	7	55.40	52.30	179.50
Trumbull County	187	161	26	(v)	55.40	76.00
Cortland	4	4	0	32.20	32.50	0.00
Girard	13	13	0	68.10	(w)	0.00
Hubbard	7	7	0	63.10	63.60	0.00
Newton Falls	4	4	0	44.90	44.90	0.00
Niles	20	19	1	64.10	62.90	100.00
Warren	66	44	22	63.60	58.20	78.00
Youngstown	0	0	0	0.00	0.00	0.00
Balance	73	70	3	52.80	52.10	(x)

°Per 1,000 live births of particular community.

Table C.10A. Premature Births Classified by Race, Number, and Rate, by County, City, and Balance of County, Ohio, 1985—Answers

County, City, and Balance of County	Premature Births	Number		Rate°		
		White	Black	Total	White	Black
Ohio	10,700	7,837	2,874	66.69	57.77	116.00
Columbia County	87	86	1	56.30	56.50	41.67
E. Liverpool	17	17	0	68.30	71.40	0.00
E. Palestine	5	5	0	66.70	66.70	0.00
Salem	10	10	0	51.00	51.50	0.00
Wellville	11	10	1	159.40	153.80	250.00
Balance	44	44	0	46.00	46.30	0.00
Mahoning County	290	153	137	78.83	54.50	157.47
Campbell	6	3	3	48.40	30.00	125.00
Canfield	6	6	0	74.10	74.10	0.00
Sebring	0	0	0	0.00	0.00	0.00
Struthers	6	5	1	41.70	36.50	142.86
Youngstown	182	56	126	112.90	67.30	157.50
Balance	90	83	7	55.40	52.30	179.50

Table C.10A. (continued)

Trumbull County	187	161	26	57.56	55.40	76.00
Cortland	4	4	0	32.20	32.50	0.00
Girard	13	13	0	68.10	71.04	0.00
Hubbard	7	7	0	63.10	63.60	0.00
Newton Falls	4	4	0	44.90	44.90	0.00
Niles	20	19	1	64.10	62.90	100.00
Warren	66	44	22	63.60	58.20	78.00
Youngstown	0	0	0	0.00	0.00	0.00
Balance	73	70	3	52.80	52.10	75.00

Table C.11. Illegitimate Births Classified by Race, Number, and Rate, by County, City, and Balance of County, Ohio, 1985

County, City, and Balance of County	Illegitimate Births	Number		Rate[°]		
		White	Black	Total	White	Black
Ohio	34,896	19,417	15,479	(y)	143.10	(z)
Columbia County	217	209	8	140.40	(aa)	333.30
E. Liverpool	64	60	4	257.00	252.10	363.10
E. Palestine	7	7	0	93.30	93.30	0.00
Salem	31	30	1	158.20	154.60	500.00
Wellville	18	16	2	260.90	246.20	500.00
Balance	97	96	1	101.40	101.10	142.90
Mahoning County	953	354	599	259.00	126.00	688.50
Campbell	30	16	14	241.90	160.00	583.30
Canfield	4	4	0	49.40	49.40	0.00
Sebring	19	19	0	263.90	263.90	0.00
Struthers	22	18	4	152.90	131.40	571.40
Youngstown	722	156	566	442.40	187.50	(bb)
Balance	156	141	15	95.90	88.80	384.60
Trumbull County	580	386	194	178.50	(cc)	567.30
Cortland	9	9	0	72.60	73.20	0.00
Girard	21	19	2	109.90	103.80	250.00
Hubbard	16	15	1	144.10	136.40	(dd)
Newton Falls	15	15	0	168.50	168.50	0.00
Niles	55	53	2	176.30	175.50	200.00
Warren	315	138	177	303.50	182.50	627.70
Youngstown	0	0	0	0.00	0.00	0.00
Balance	149	137	12	107.70	102.00	300.00

[°]Per 1,000 live births of particular community

Table C.11A. Illegitimate Births Classified by Race, Number, and Rate, by County, City, and Balance of County, Ohio, 1985—Answers

County, City, and Balance of County	Illegitimate Births	Number		Rate°		
		White	Black	Total	White	Black
Ohio	34,896	19,417	15,479	217.51	143.10	624.98
Columbia County	217	209	8	140.40	137.32	333.30
E. Liverpool	64	60	4	257.00	252.10	363.10
E. Palestine	7	7	0	93.30	93.30	0.00
Salem	31	30	1	158.20	154.60	500.00
Wellville	18	16	2	260.90	246.20	500.00
Balance	97	96	1	101.40	101.10	142.90
Mahoning County	953	354	599	259.00	126.00	688.50
Campbell	30	16	14	241.90	160.00	583.30
Canfield	4	4	0	49.40	49.40	0.00
Sebring	19	19	0	263.90	263.90	0.00
Struthers	22	18	4	152.90	131.40	571.40
Youngstown	722	156	566	442.40	187.50	707.50
Balance	156	141	15	95.90	88.80	384.60
Trumbull County	580	386	194	178.50	132.78	567.30
Cortland	9	9	0	72.60	73.20	0.00
Girard	21	19	2	109.90	103.80	250.00
Hubbard	16	15	1	144.10	136.40	1,000.00
Newton Falls	15	15	0	168.50	168.50	0.00
Niles	55	53	2	176.30	175.50	200.00
Warren	315	138	177	303.50	182.50	627.70
Youngstown	0	0	0	0.00	0.00	0.00
Balance	149	137	12	107.70	102.00	300.00

Rationale for Problems for Tables C.9–C.11

Table C.9

To figure item (a), divide total live births in Ohio (160,433) by the total Ohio population (10,797,630) times 1,000 (base).

Item (b): 1,546/113,572 × 1,000
Item (c): 249/16,687 × 1,000
Item (d): 957/73,615 × 1,000
Item (e): 3,679/289,487 × 1,000
Item (f): 124/11,619 × 1,000
Item (g): 1,612/115,427 × 1,000
Item (h): 1,626/138,204 × 1,000

Item (i): 3,249/241,863 × 1,000
Item (j): 124/5,011 × 1,000
Item (k): 89/4,960 × 1,000
Item (l): 1,038/56,629 × 1,000
Item (m): 1,383/130,404 × 1,000

Table C.10

To figure item (n), divide 10,700 by 160,433 live births times 1,000. Premature birth rate is the number of premature births per 1,000 live births. There were almost 11,000 premature births within the total number of births (160,433).

Item (o): 7,837/135,666 × 1,000
Item (p): 1/24 × 1,000. There was 1.00 nonwhite premature birth in Columbia County among the 24 nonwhite live births.
Item (q): 290/3,679 × 1,000
Item (r): 137/870 × 1,000
Item (s): 1.00/7 × 1,000
Item (t): 182/1,612 × 1,000
Item (u): 126/800 × 1,000
Item (v): 187/3,249 × 1,000
Item (w): 13/183 × 1,000
Item (x): 3/40 × 1,000

Table C.11

To figure item (y), divide 34,896 by 160,433 live births times 1,000. This is the rate of total illegitimate births per 1,000 live births. There was a total of 34,896 illegitimate births in the state of Ohio among the 160,433 live births.

Item (z): 15,479/24,767 × 1,000
Item (aa): 209/1,522 × 1,000
Item (bb): 566/800 × 1,000
Item (cc): 386/2,907 × 1,000
Item (dd): 1.00/1.00 × 1,000

Appendix D
Basic Mathematics: A Review

Some of you may not have had a basic math course since junior high school. For those of you who have had a college statistics course, you might remember that you really didn't need a working knowledge of basic math as statistics is primarily conceptual in nature. In vital statistics, however, it is important to be comfortable using math. True, the type of math is relatively basic, but it can be frustrating and difficult if you haven't had to use such skills for a number of years. The purpose of this appendix is to refresh your basic math skills. Obviously, if you feel comfortable with basic math, you can skip this section.

It is somewhat ironic that I am writing on basic math. Math was never my strong area. In the seventh and eighth grades I managed C's in my math classes. Then an error directed me to algebra in the ninth grade and my sheer panic soon turned to great joy. Probably the best teacher I have ever had in my life (James Silgen) taught my algebra class. I shocked myself and earned straight A's. I was so excited about math that I signed up for geometry in the tenth grade, with a long-term plan to go to college to become a math teacher.

Three weeks into my tenth-grade geometry class I crashed. I was so far behind, bewildered, and dismayed that I dropped geometry. So I have never taken a formal math class since ninth grade. My high school (grades ten to twelve) never required me to take a math class for graduation, and I attended a college that also did not require a math class. My graduate programs (both the master's and the doctorate) obviously didn't require any math classes, either, but they did require statistics. In the five statistics courses I completed in my graduate program, I earned straight A's.

I'm telling you this story not to pat myself on the back (although at times I am surprised at how well I have done in statistics without any math classes) but to illustrate that you don't need math skills to successfully complete a statistics class. Again, statistics is mostly conceptual, and anyone these days who does the work by hand is taking the hard route. Yet I use math now all of the time; a professor of mine once said that somewhere, somehow, I learned these basic math skills. (Perhaps the fact that I was a long-distance runner constantly trying to convert miles into kilometers could account for this.) Nonetheless, I have learned and utilize these basic skills.

For a vital statistician to be truly competent, he or she needs to feel confident in using basic math skills. Thus, this appendix will focus on the following basic skills: fractions, decimals, and percentages.

Before we start, I will present a quick review of the various signs used in basic math computations:

+	Plus—indicates addition
−	Minus—indicates subtraction
×	Multiplied by—indicates multiplication (sometimes the × is replaced by an asterisk °)
/	Divided by—indicates division (also ÷)
=	Equal to—indicates equality
[ ], ( ), { }	Brackets, parentheses, or braces. They all mean the same. In math, one performs all computations within these signs before computations outside the signs.
Σ	Summation of—Σ (x + y) means to find the sum of x added to y.
.	Decimal point—used following a whole number. All numbers to the right of the decimal point are a part of a whole number.
10^x	Indicates the power to which a number is raised ($10^2 = 10 \times 10 = 100$)
: :: :	Indicates proportion (5:10 :: 20:40)

The following are some terms you should also know:

Numerator—the number above the line in a fraction
Denominator—the number below the line in a fraction
Dividend—the number that is being divided (in both of these examples, the dividend is 21: 3)$\overline{21}$ 21 ÷ 3)
Divisor—the number that divides (in the above examples, the divisor is 3)

Fractions

Fractions are made up of two parts. The part above the line is called the *numerator*, and the part below the line is called the *denominator*. When the value of the fraction is less than one, it is called a proper fraction. Improper fractions are those fractions that have a value greater than one (the numerator is larger than the denominator). Finally, a mixed number is one that combines a whole number and a fraction. To add more confusion to the mess, there are complex fractions. These are fractions that have additional fractions in either the numerator and/or the denominator.

Proper fraction	1/2
Improper fraction	4/2
Mixed fraction	1 1/2
Complex fraction	$\dfrac{2}{2/4}$

A unique rule with fractions is that as long as you multiply or divide the numerator and the denominator by the same number, the value remains the same. For example, suppose you have the fraction 1/2 (one-half). As long as the bottom number is twice that of the top number, it means the same as 1/2. So:

$$\frac{1 \times 10}{2 \times 10} = \frac{10}{20}$$

or

$$\frac{10 \div 10}{20 \div 10} = \frac{1}{2}$$

Usually, when you are dealing with fractions, you want to use them in the lowest terms. This means that you have reduced the numerator and the denominator as far as possible without changing the value of the fraction. The lowest term of 100/200 is 1/2. To find the lowest term, you divide the numerator and the denominator by the largest number that both can be divided by. Sometimes you need to repeat this step several times. For example, to reduce 200/400, you may first divide both by 100 to get 2/4. You can then reduce 2/4 by dividing both by 2 to get 1/2. If you don't know where to start, first check to see if both the numerator and the denominator are even numbers. If they are, you can start by dividing them by 2.

There may be times in which you'll need to raise the fraction to a higher term. Again, you can do that by multiplying both the numerator and the denominator by the same number. For example:

$$\frac{1 \times 10}{2 \times 10} = \frac{10}{20}$$

If you have an improper fraction, you can convert it to a mixed number by dividing the numerator by the denominator and then placing the remainder over the denominator. Thus, to convert 23/6, you would divide 23 by 6 to equal 3 5/6. To convert a mixed number to an improper fraction, multiply the denominator times the whole number and then add the numerator. That new number is the numerator; the denominator remains the same. For example:

$$4\ 2/3 = 14/3\ (3 \times 4 = 12 + 2 = 14)$$

If you need to add fractions that have different denominators, you need to first convert all fractions into common fractions (fractions with common denominators). The easiest way I find to do this is to multiply the two denominators. You then need to recalculate both numerators. For example, in 1/2 + 3/4 the common denominator is eight. You'll need to multiply the numerators by 4 and 2 respectively. So, 1/2 + 3/4 = 4/8 + 6/8 = 10/8. You then need to convert 10/8 to its lowest term (10/8 = 1 2/8), which can be reduced further to 1 1/4. There are quicker ways to do this, but I'm trying to stick to a certain procedure.

To subtract fractions, you also need to convert both denominators into common numbers. Thus, to figure 5/6 − 1/3, you need to convert both denominators to 18: 5/6 = 15/18 and 1/3 = 6/18: 15/18 − 6/18 = 9/18 = 1/2.

To multiply fractions by whole numbers, simply multiply the whole number by the numerator. For instance, 5 × 1/2 = 5 × 1/2 = 5/2 = 2 1/2.

To divide a fraction by a whole number, simply multiply the whole number by the denominator. Remember that you invert the divisor in division and multiply the numbers. For example, 1/2 ÷ 5 = 1/2 ÷ 5/1 = 1/2 × 1/5 = 1/10.

To multiply one fraction by another fraction, multiply the numerators and the denominators and then reduce to the lowest term. For example, 2/3 × 1/2 = 2/6 = 1/3.

To multiply mixed numbers, change the mixed number to an improper fraction, multiply, and reduce accordingly. For example, 2 1/2 × 3 1/3 = 5/2 × 10/3 = 50/6 = 8 2/6 = 8 1/3.

To divide a whole number or a fraction by a fraction, you must invert the divisor and multiply. For example, 2/3 ÷ 1/4 = 2/3 × 4/1 = 8/3 = 2 2/3.

Decimals

Decimals are commonly used in vital statistics. A decimal is a part of a whole number and is placed to the right of the decimal point. For example, in 12.34, the 34 is in the decimal area.

The decimal point is the start of the decimal range. Each column of a digit represents a certain amount. For example, .1 is in the first place of a decimal and is read "one-tenth"; .4 is read "four-tenths"; and .4 is the same as 4/10.

Place of Digit	*Pronunciation*	*Example*
First decimal point	Tenths	.4
Second decimal point	Hundredths	.04
Third decimal point	Thousandths	.004
Fourth decimal point	Ten thousandths	.0004
Fifth decimal point	Hundred thousandths	.00004
Sixth decimal point	Millionth	.000004

To change any common fraction into a decimal, divide the numerator by the denominator. For example, 7/8 = .875.

Keep in mind that .1 and .10 mean the same thing. Also, .1 is equal to .10000000000. The decimal place basically indicates that this decimal is 1/10 of something. This concept is very important when you add decimals: make sure that the decimal points align. For example, here are the right and wrong ways to add decimals:

Right	Wrong
125.905	125.905
55.800	55.800
1.155	1.155
182.860	

To multiply decimals, proceed as if they are whole numbers. At the conclusion, add the number of decimal places that are included in the numbers multiplied to your final answer. For example:

```
   5.25    (two decimal places)
   2.55    (two decimal places)
 13.3875  (four decimal places)
```

To multiply a decimal by ten, a hundred, a thousand, ten thousand, etc., simply move the decimal place to the right as many spaces as there are zeroes in your multiplier. For example:

```
5.25 × 10   =   52.5
5.25 × 100  =   525.0
5.25 × 1000 = 5250.0
```

On the other hand, to divide a decimal by ten, a hundred, etc., move the decimal place to the left as many spaces as there are zeroes in your divisor. For example:

```
5.25 ÷ 10   = .52500
5.25 ÷ 100  = .05250
5.25 ÷ 1000 = .00525
```

To divide a decimal by a whole number, complete the task as though no decimal is present. After completing, place the decimal point directly above the decimal point in the dividend. For example:

$$
\begin{array}{r}
12.25 \\
2\overline{)\,24.50}
\end{array}
$$

To divide a decimal by a decimal, move the decimal point of the divisor to the end of the number. In the dividend, move the decimal point the same number of spaces. You may need to add zeros to the dividend to complete the task. For example:

$$222.2 \div 10.5 = 10.5\overline{)\,222.2} = 105.\overline{)\,2222}$$

or

$$25 \div 10.5 = 10.5\overline{)25} = 105\overline{)\,250}$$

Rounding off decimals is done quite frequently. At what decimal place you decide to round off is up to you and the point that you are trying to make. You can round up (or down) depending on the last digit in the number. The key number to rounding up or down is 5. If that last number is 5, you can round up to the next highest number; if it is 4 or less, you round down to the next lowest number. For example:

```
.55 =  .60
.54 =  .50
.09 =  .10
1.01 = 1.00
```

If you want to round off a large decimal to only two places, then just look at the third number and round up/down accordingly.

```
.78843 = .79
.788   = .79
```

Finally, you can convert a decimal to a fraction by simply putting the number over the place represented in the decimal. For example:

.6   = 6/10
.06   = 6/100
.875 = 875/1,000

After that, you can then reduce it to its lowest term.

Percentages

A percentage means 1/100 of something: thus, 1% is 1/100; 50% means 50/100 (or one-half). Keep in mind that .05 is the same as 5%. To complicate matters further, you can have a decimal in a percentage. For example, .055 is the same as 5.5%.

To convert a decimal to a percentage, simply move the decimal to the right by two places. For example:

.08 is 8%
.80 is 80%
.85 is 85%
.005 is .5%

On the other hand, to change a percentage to a decimal, simply move the decimal to the left by two places. For example:

 8% = .08
80% = .80
85% = .85
 .5% = .005

Remember that .05 is not the same as .05%. The first number states 5 out of 100, whereas the second indicates 5 out of 10,000.

Problems you may be asked to solve:

1. Find the percentage of a particular number.
    What is 20% of 500?
    20% = .20
    Multiply: 500 × .20 = 100

    Answer: 100 is 20% of 500

    Another way to determine this is to cross-multiply. You need to first set it up as follows:

    20% is the same as 20/100
    You need to find the x of 500:

$$\frac{20}{100} = \frac{x}{500}$$

Cross-multiplying gives you $20 \times 500 \div 100 = 10,000 \div 100 = 100$.

2. Find what percentage a number is of another.
   150 is what percentage of 300?

$$\frac{150}{300} = \frac{1}{2} = 50\%$$

Answer: 150 is 50% of 300

3. Find a number when a percentage of that number is known.
   100 is 20% of what number?
   20% = 1/5
   $100 \div 1/5 = 100 \times 5/1 = 500$

Answer: 100 is 20% of 500

If you use the cross-multiplication process, it would work as follows:

20% = 20/100
100 is part of x

$$\frac{20}{100} = \frac{100}{x} =$$

$100 \times 100 = 10,000 \div 20 = 500$

Math Problems

The following are practice problems for you to solve (the answers can be found below).

1. 1/2 + 4/5 =
2. 1/2 + 3/5 =
3. 1/2 + 4/9 =
4. 3/8 + 5/6 =
5. 1/8 + 5/6 =
6. 1/4 + 2/3 =
7. 1/3 + 3/8 =
8. 3/4 + 3/5 =
9. 4/5 + 7/9 =
10. 5/6 − 5/8 =
11. 2/3 − 3/5 =
12. 3/4 − 5/12 =
13. 2/5 − 1/8 =
14. 5/6 − 4/5 =
15. 3/5 − 5/9 =
16. 3/5 ÷ 5 =
17. 1/9 × 3/5 =
18. 6 × 1/9 =
19. 3/8 ÷ 6 =

20. 2/5 × 25 =
21. 5 × 1/3 =
22. 2/3 ÷ 3 =
23. 5/6 × 30 =
24. 2/3 × 3/4 =
25. 3/4 ÷ 12 =
26. 1/3 × 3/8 =
27. 3 × 3/4 =
28. 1/3 × 1/4 × 1/2 × 3/4 =
29. 3/4 × 5/8 × 1/5 × 2/3 =
30. 2/5 × 3/8 × 1/2 × 8/8 =
31. 3/7 × 3/5 =
32. 3/8 × 2/3 =
33. 2/15 × 4/21 × 7/8 × 5 =
34. 14/15 × 9/12 =
35. 3/8 × 12 =
36. 5/6 × 5/9 =
37. 15/16 × 7/90 =
38. 7/27 × 9/14 =

39. 18 + 1/2 =
40. 3/5 + 1/15 =
41. 2/3 ÷ 1/2 =
42. 4/7 ÷ 1/8 =
43. 1 2/3 × 3/4 =
44. 2 1/2 × 1 3/4 =
45. 3 1/2 × 1/4 =
46. 1 1/8 ÷ 3/16 =
47. 2/3 + 1/4 + 1/2 =
48. (2/3 ÷ 1/5) ÷ (1/4 × 1/3) =
49. (2 1/2 + 3 1/3) ÷ (4 + 2/3) =
50. 18.5 × 4 =
51. 3.9 × 2.4 =
52. 45 × .72 =
53. 143 × .214 =
54. .56 × .74 =

55. .224 × .302 =
56. 9.06 × .045 =
57. .008 × 751.1 =
58. 8.7 × 10 =
59. .0069 × 10 =
60. 492.568 ÷ 1,000 =
61. 534.79 ÷ 100 =
62. .07156 ÷ 1,000 =
63. 25% of 256 =
64. 30% of 600 =
65. 1/2% of 500 =
66. 12 1/2% of 96 =
67. 12 is 25% of what number?
68. 8 is 2 1/2% of what number?
69. 1/2 is what percent of 2/3?

Answers to Math Problems

1. 1/2 + 4/5 = 5/10 + 8/10 = 13/10 = 1 3/10
2. 1/2 + 3/5 = 5/10 + 6/10 = 11/10 = 1 1/10
3. 1/2 + 4/9 = 9/18 + 8/18 = 17/18
4. 3/8 + 5/6 = 18/48 + 40/48 = 58/48 = 1 10/48 = 1 5/24
   (You must reduce 10/48; so divide both the numerator and the denominator by 2 to get the final product.)
5. 1/8 + 5/6 = 6/48 + 40/48 = 46/48 = 23/24
6. 1/4 + 2/3 = 3/12 + 8/12 = 11/12
7. 1/3 + 3/8 = 8/24 + 9/24 = 17/24
8. 3/4 + 3/5 = 15/20 + 12/20 = 27/20 = 1 7/20
9. 4/5 + 7/9 = 36/45 + 35/45 = 71/45 = 1 36/45 = 1 4/5
   (You must reduce 36/45: divide each by 9 to get 4/5.)
10. 5/6 − 5/8 = 40/48 − 30/48 = 10/48 = 5/24
11. 2/3 − 3/5 = 10/15 − 9/15 = 1/15
12. 3/4 − 5/12 = 9/12 − 5/12 = 4/12 = 1/3
13. 2/5 − 1/8 = 16/40 − 5/40 = 11/40
14. 5/6 − 4/5 = 25/30 − 24/30 = 1/30
15. 3/5 − 5/9 = 27/45 − 25/45 = 2/45
16. 3/5 ÷ 5 = 3/5 ÷ 5/1 = 3/5 × 1/5 = 4/25
17. 1/9 × 3/5 = 3/45 = 1/15
18. 6 × 1/9 = 6/9 = 2/3
19. 3/8 ÷ 6 = 3/8 ÷ 6/1 = 3/8 × 1/6 = 3/48 = 1/16
20. 2/5 × 25 = 2/5 × 25/1 = 50/5 = 10
21. 5 × 1/3 = 5/1 × 1/3 = 5/3 = 1 2/3
22. 2/3 ÷ 3 = 2/3 ÷ 3/1 = 2/3 × 1/3 = 2/9
23. 5/6 × 30 = 5/6 × 30/1 = 150/6 = 25
24. 2/3 × 3/4 = 6/12 = 1/2
25. 3/4 ÷ 12 = 3/4 ÷ 12/1 = 3/4 × 1/12 = 3/48 = 1/16
26. 1/3 × 3/8 = 3/24 = 1/8

27. $3 \times 3/4 = 3/1 \times 3/4 = 9/4 = 2\ 1/4$
28. $1/3 \times 1/4 \times 1/2 \times 3/4 = 3/96 = 1/32$
29. $3/4 \times 5/8 \times 1/5 \times 2/3 = 30/480 = 1/16$
30. $2/5 \times 3/8 \times 1/2 \times 8/8 = 48/640 \times 3/40$
31. $3/7 \times 3/5 = 9/35$
32. $3/8 \times 2/3 = 6/24 = 1/4$
33. $2/15 \times 4/21 \times 7/8 \times 5 = 2/15 \times 4/21 \times 7/8 \times 5/1 = 280/2,520 = 1/9$
34. $14/15 \times 9/12 = 126/180 = 64/90 = 32/45$
35. $3/8 \times 12 = 3/8 \times 12/1 = 36/8 = 4\ 4/8 = 4\ 1/2$
36. $5/6 + 5/9 = 25/54$
37. $15/16 \times 7/90 = 105/1,440 = 5/72$
38. $7/27 \times 9/14 = 63/378 = 1/6$
39. $18 + 1/2 = 18\ 1/2$
40. $3/5 + 1/15 = 9/15 + 1/15 = 10/15 = 2/3$
41. $2/3 \div 1/2 = 2/3 \times 2/1 = 4/3 = 1\ 1/34$
42. $4/7 \div 1/8 = 4/7 \times 8/1 = 32/7 = 4\ 5/7$
43. $1\ 2/3 \times 3/4 = 5/3 \times 3/4 = 15/12 = 1\ 3/12 = 1\ 1/4$
44. $2\ 1/2 \times 1\ 3/4 = 5/2 \times 7/4 = 35/8 = 4\ 3/8$
45. $3\ 1/2 \times 1/4 = 7/2 \times 1/4 = 7/8$
46. $1\ 1/8 \div 3/16 = 9/8 \div 3/16 = 9/8 \times 16/3 = 144/24 = 6$
47. $2/3 + 1/4 = 1/2 = 8/12 + 3/12 + 6/12 = 17/12 = 1\ 5/12$
48. $(2/3 \div 1/5) \div (1/4 \times 1/3) =$
    $(2/3 \times 5/1) \div (1/4 \times 1/3) =$
    $10/3 \div 1/12 = 10/3 \times 12/1 = 120/3 = 40$
49. $(2\ 1/2 + 3\ 1/3) \div (4 + 2/3) =$
    $(5/2 + 10/3) \div (4\ 2/3) =$
    $(15/6 + 20/6) \div 14/3 =$
    $35/6 \div 14/3 = 35/6 \times 3/14 = 105/84 = 1\ 21/105$
50. $18.5 \times 4 = 74.0$
51. $3.9 \times 2.4 = 9.36$
52. $45 \times .72 = 32.40$
53. $143 \times .214 = 30.602$
54. $.56 \times .74 = .4144$
55. $.224 \times .302 = .067648$
56. $9.06 \times .045 = .407700$
57. $.008 \times 751.1 = 6.00880000$
58. $8.7 \times 10 = 87$
59. $.0069 \times 10 = .069$
60. $492.568 \div 1,000 = 492,568/1,000 \div 1,000 =$
    $492,568/1,000 \div 1,000/1 =$
    $492,568/1,000 \times 1/1,000 =$
    $492,568/1,000,000 = .492568$
61. $534.79 \div 100 = 53,479/100 \div 100 =$
    $53,479/100 \div 100/1 =$
    $53,479/100 \times 1/100 =$
    $53,479/10,000 = 5.3479$
62. $.07156 \div 1,000 = 7,156/100,000 \div 1,000/1 =$

    7,156/100,000 × 1/1,000 =

    7,156/100,000,000 = .00007156

63. 25% of 256 = 25/100 × x/256 =

    (25 × 256) ÷ 100 =

    6,400 ÷ 100 = 64

    64 is 25% of 256

    (You must cross-multiply to find x.)

64. 30% of 600 = 30/100 × x/600 =

    (30 × 600) ÷ 100 = 1,800 ÷ 100 = 180

    180 is 30% of 600

65. 1/2% of 500 is what?

    .5/100 × x/500 = .5 × 500 ÷ 100 = 2.5

    2.5 is 1/2% of 500

66. 12 1/2% of 96 is what?

    12.5/100 × x/96 =

    12.5 × 96 ÷ 100 = 12

    12 is 12 1/2% of 96

67. 12 is 25% of what number?

    12/x × 25/100 = 12 × 100 ÷ 25 = 48

    12 is 25% of 48

68. 8 is 2 1/2% of what number?

    8/x × 2.5/100 = 8 × 100 ÷ 2.5 = 320

    8 is 2 1/2% of 320

69. 1/2 is what percent of 2/3?

    1/2 ÷ 2/3 = x/100

    1/2 × 3/2 = x/100

    3/4 = x/100

    x = 75

    1/2 is 75% of 2/3

Index

abortion, definition of, 1
adjusting, direct method of, 57
Apgar score, definition of, 2
Atlas, U.S., 8

chi-square, 19
Clements, John, 8
Comprehensive Look at Illinois Today, County by County, A, 8
Consolidated Metropolitan Statistical Area (CMSA), 2
correlations, 16, 18; negative, 17; positive, 17

data, 9; analysis of, 11; demographic, 1; interval, 9, 14; nominal, 9, 13; ordinal, 9, 13; ratio, 9, 14
deaths: expected, 58; fetal definition of, 3
decision tree, 68–69
deviation, standard, 14–16
difference: absolute, 27; relative, 27

graph, 24; abscissa, 24; axes of, 24; bar, 25; definition of, 24; histogram, 24; line, 24; ordinate, 24; pie, 26

Illinois Project for Local Assessment of Needs (IPLAN), The, 7
infant, definition of: death, 3; full-term, 3; live birth, 3; neonatal death, 3; perinatal death, 3; premature, 3

mean, 12–13
median, 12, 13
mode, 11, 13
morbidity, 3

National Ambulatory Medical Care Survey, 7
National Center for Health Statistics, 6; *Vital Statistics of the United States*, 6; *Vital Statistics Report*, 6
National Death Index, 7
National Health and Nutrition Examination Survey, 7
National Health Interview Survey, 7
National Hospital Discharge Survey, 8
National Inventory of Family Planning Service, 8
National Master Facility Inventory, 8
National Medical Care Utilization and Expenditures, 8
National Mortality Survey, 8
National Natality Survey, 7
National Nursing Home Survey, 8
National Reporting System for Family Planning, 8

PCUSA (computer program), 8
Pearson Product, 18
population: enumerated, 54, 55; pooled, 55, 56, 58; standard, 54
Primary Metropolitan Statistical Area (PMSA), 2
proportion, 34

range, 14
rate: adjusted, 42; age-specific, 43; base, 40; crude, 42; definition, 41; fertility, 42; formula, 42; incidence, 43, 44; prevalence, 43; specific, 43; standardized, 54; standardizing, 57; types, 42
ratio, 33

sensitivity, 63
significance, 20
specificity, 64

Mark J. Kittleson, Ph.D., is an associate professor of health education at Southern Illinois University at Carbondale, where he teaches vital statistics, research design, and evaluation of health programs. He has published over forty peer-reviewed research projects and has presented over seventy research papers at a variety of professional conferences including the American Public Health Association. He is a fellow of the Association for Advancement of Health Education.